Supremely Wrong sets the record straight while delivering hope and healing to those impacted by the scourge of abortion.

Dr. Alveda C. King
Evangelist, Civil Rights for the Unborn
Niece of Rev. Dr. Martin Luther King, Jr.

Dr. Brent Boles has written a medically informed and deeply challenging book about the nature of the abortion debate, and why—nearly five decades after *Roe v. Wade*—it is the most contentious and portentous clash facing the nation. *Supremely Wrong* is a must-read on an issue that will not and cannot go away.

Chuck Donovan
President, Charlotte Lozier Institute

Have you ever felt helpless when trying to explain your thoughts on abortion? The divisions in our culture's life-and-death battle deepen daily. Arm yourself with the knowledge necessary to not only stand up for life, but feel comfortable while doing it. This book by Dr. Brent Boles is filled with facts and expert medical information essential for defending the most important issue of our time—life.

Sue Thayer
Director of Outreach, 40 Days for Life
Former Clinic Manager, Planned Parenthood of the Heartland (Iowa)

More inspired and detailed than any pro-life handbook to date, *Supremely Wrong* will be a treasure for the entire movement. Dr. Brent Boles leverages his unique personal experiences in the fields of medical practice and legislation to reveal a clear roadmap to the future in America.

Matt Lockett
Executive Director, Bound4LIFE International
Author, *The Dream King* and *Prayer That Impacts the World*

In his book, *Supremely Wrong: The Injustice of Abortion*, Dr. Brent Boles removes the veil on all things related to both sides of the abortion issue. No one can plead ignorance any longer.

Victoria Robinson
Author and Speaker
Director of External Relations, Save the Storks

What impresses me about Dr. Boles isn't his credentials as a physician— it's his love for truth grounded in medical ethics. This book provides new insights into why and how we must defend every precious life.

Harry R. Jackson Jr.
Senior Pastor, Hope Christian Church
Bishop, Ambassadors of Hope

SUPREMELY

THE INJUSTICE OF ABORTION

WRONG

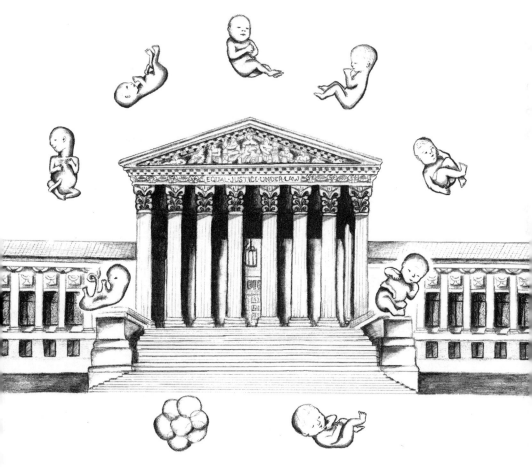

BRENT BOLES, M.D.

Published by NEWTYPE Publishing

ISBN: 978-1-949709-77-3
eISBN: 978-1-949709-80-3

Printed in the United States.

TABLE OF CONTENTS

INTRODUCTION

There is perhaps no greater divide in America today than the divide between those who celebrate *Roe v. Wade* and those who mourn it. Gallup polls[1] over the past forty years consistently show Americans come down nearly equal on the question of how they self-identify; in late 2018, the figures were 48 percent "pro-life" and 48 percent "pro-choice."

As I sat in Labor and Delivery one day several years ago, I became aware of the fact that that particular date was the 35th anniversary of *Roe v Wade*. For the remainder of that day, I worked intermittently to write my thoughts. It was a busy day. With one young mother about to deliver her first child and another patient of mine who had just arrived in early labor, I was struck once again by just how far the Supreme Court missed the mark with that decision.

When the Supremes handed down their decision, the only evidence of independent life in the unborn child they had to consider was the mother's perception of the baby's movement. We now have very different technology—technology that demonstrates early life as soon as a couple of weeks after conception. We can detect the hormonal evidence of that life with a blood test before the mother (not mother-to-be) is even late for her menstrual period. We can see a heart beating within the early fetal pole as early as three weeks after conception. This is life…and while it certainly is not *independent* of its mother's life, it is most definitely *distinct* from the mother's life.

Dr. Keith Moore's classic textbook on embryology, used in almost all medical school classes on human development, refers to the single-celled zygote and says "The cell results from fertilization of an oocyte by a sperm and is the beginning of a human being."[2] Dr. Bradley M. Patten's textbook *Human Embryology* says that fertilization "marks the initiation of the life of a new individual."[3] There is no real scientific uncertainty about when life begins—and even if there were, the benefit of the doubt should go to the preservation of life.

What is the real and practical difference between the newborn I was about to deliver and a walking, talking two-year-old toddler? The most fundamental and essential difference is two years. That's right—time only. There are other things to which most people would point as obvious differences, but consider this: each and every difference between a newborn and that same child as a walking, talking toddler is the result of the passage of time. What is the most fundamental difference between the four weeks post-conception fetal pole and the newborn in the warmer? The passage of time. Any and all differences to which one can point in an attempt to make a distinction between the fetus and the newborn are the result of the passage of time. The act of ending the life of a toddler, or even of the newborn on the warmer, is indisputably murder—yet our laws allow the daily destruction of the lives of unborn children who have simply not yet lived long enough to cry, mess a diaper, or walk into the room and enthusiastically yell, "Daddy!" when daddy gets home from work.

So here we are—in a situation where political correctness reigns supreme over simple correctness and accuracy. We are told: It's a choice, not a child. It's unfortunate, but choice is a right and it must be protected. Millions of women will die in back alleys if they don't have the right to choose. What about the more than sixty million who have died in operating rooms and clinics, mostly for the sake of convenience? The Nazis killed six million innocent Jews for what they perceived to be the sake of convenience—we in this country have killed more than ten times that many babies. If advocates for the pro-choice movement only had the spine to acknowledge, with truth and accuracy, exactly what abortion really is, it wouldn't sound so politically correct and inoffensive. Here's a news flash: Sometimes the truth is offensive!

Let's consider truth for a minute. What the vast majority of Americans don't realize is that the lawyers who argued the cases *Roe v. Wade* and *Doe v. Bolton* both lied to the Supreme Court. They misrepresented the facts of the cases to the justices. It's true—what far too many Americans consider to be nearly sacred court precedents were based on lies. The material facts of the cases and the actual circumstances of the petitioners were misrepresented to the justices. Isn't the pursuit of truth supposed to be the underlying bedrock principle of our court system?

We have become a nation that is truly double-minded about our children. A woman with a child that delivers at twenty-five weeks at home unexpectedly—then decides to put the living child in a bag and throw it in the dumpster—will be tried for murder. A woman who chooses to go see a late-term abortionist at twenty-five weeks can have him administer some sort of poison to the child and then induce labor, so a dead child be delivered, or have the abortionist perform some sort of dismemberment procedure on the living child. To the pro-choice movement, she has bravely chosen an option that the law allows and is seen as a hero to have it done.

Our venerable House of Representatives, with its many pro-choice members, unanimously voted in the year 2000 to make it illegal to execute a pregnant woman. The only reason for such a vote is the recognition that the preborn child is a living individual with the right to live because he is distinct from his mother.[4] That same House of Representatives has many members who regard the "right to choose" as a literal sacrament supposedly protected by the Constitution's "right to privacy." Let's consider the implications. That "right to privacy" doesn't allow me, as a doctor, to help a woman plan the murder of a cheating, abusive spouse, but it allows the relationship between a doctor and patient to plan the termination of a pregnancy. Do you see the double-mindedness?

More than half of the people who find themselves reading this are the result of an unplanned pregnancy. If you were born after the Supreme Court ruling in 1973, you are breathing today because your mother chose to have you. You would most certainly say that she chose well. Those whose mothers chose differently than yours have no voice with which to protest.

In the time it took for me to finish this original writing several years ago, a little bit at a time, I delivered both of the patients of whom I spoke in the opening paragraph. One handsome little boy, and one beautiful little girl. Neither one planned, but both wanted...and each one here simply because their mothers chose well. That which follows in this work is the result of several more years of study, thought, and activism on this issue, and is intended for two audiences. It is my hope that my words have been assembled in a way that those who read will find persuasive.

Those who believe that a woman's right to choose is of prime importance, but who are willing to consider the subsequent material in this book, will find their worldview challenged. Those who believe in the sanctity of life will, upon complete consideration of this work, find themselves better prepared to participate in this gargantuan struggle in a meaningful and successful manner.

CHAPTER 1

UNDERSTANDING WHEN LIFE BEGINS

In the quest to understand the discourse about abortion, it is best to start at the beginning in order to grasp all that one must. Those in America who have expended so much effort to convince us all that abortion is good, just, moral, and necessary all have one commonality. They ignore the question of when life begins.

In an interview with Cecile Richards, who at the time was president of Planned Parenthood, news anchor Jorge Ramos tried twice to get her to answer the question: "When does life begin?" She steadfastly avoided his queries and deflected the conversation back to her talking points. Among other responses, she said, "I don't know that it's really relevant to the conversation." In a different interview, with Playboy magazine, she avoided multiple times answering the question in a meaningful way. She said, "It depends on the pregnancy." Then she claimed to have spoken to doctors who informed her that, "There is no specific moment when life begins." She was asked, "Is there any point during pregnancy when an abortion would be terminating a life?" To that question she replied, "That's a question medical folks have dealt with, and I'm not a doctor. I've spent a lot of time with OB-GYNs, and they will tell you there is no specific moment when life begins." Her answers, like the answers of any abortion activist when challenged on these issues, are deceptive subterfuge.

I would submit to you that the question of when life begins is not only important; it is the most relevant question in this conversation. Any statement that indicates that we cannot know when life begins is demonstrably false. In the pages that follow, I will introduce in layman's terms some basic medical understanding of human reproduction. Even if such frank descriptions seem to go "over your head" or make you squeamish as a non-medical professional, I encourage you not to rush through this chapter. Anyone seeking to engage in serious public dialogue on human life issues must have a firm grasp of the basics.

Embryology is the branch of science that studies human development. All medical schools in America must teach an embryology course, one that most students take during the very first year of medical school. It is a foundational subject, vital to understanding human anatomy and physiology. To those students who wish to pursue careers in obstetrics, pediatrics, or surgery, it is particularly important. All medical students must obtain a passing grade in this course. Virtually all medical schools in America use one or the other of two classic textbooks on embryology. Dr. Keith Moore wrote *The Developing Human: Clinically Oriented Embryology,* and Dr. Bradley M. Patten wrote *Human Embryology.* These books pin down the moment that life begins with no ambiguity whatsoever. In the first chapter of his book, Dr. Moore discusses the zygote, which is the single-celled human that briefly exists after fertilization until it begins to divide and the cells multiply. About the zygote, Dr. Keith Moore says: "The cell results from fertilization of an oocyte by a sperm and is the beginning of a human being."[5] Dr. Patten agrees with Dr. Moore's statement as to when life begins and says in the first chapter of his book that conception "marks the initiation of the life of a new individual." [6]

So much for the "ambiguity" surrounding the point at which life begins! Consider the question another way: If the pregnancy has not produced a living child, why is an abortion procedure needed to end the pregnancy? Isn't the only reason the administration of an abortifacient drug or the performance of an abortive procedure is needed is that there *is* a living child? Indeed, a child will deliver soon thereafter if the pregnancy remains uninterrupted. If life hasn't begun, why must it be killed when it is unwanted? You can only kill that which is alive; and that which is not alive does not need killing.

The mechanics of human reproduction are well known and understood. The facts of embryology cited above have been taught to all doctors in America for decades, including the OB/GYNs to whom Ms. Richards referred. There is no debate about how it happens. Even more significantly, doctors are taught how to assess the microscopic developing human for signs of life at even the earliest stages of pregnancy. Multiple medical texts, as well as instructions from the American College of Obstetrics and Gynecology, teach us how to determine the viability of the pregnancy as early as two or three weeks after conception.

Conception is the moment at which a single sperm enters a single egg. It is at that moment that twenty-three single chromosomes from the mother join twenty-three single chromosomes from the father. This micro-explosion immediately produces a combination of genetic traits and attributes which is not only undeniably human, but also irrefutably unique. The particular combination which then exists has never existed before and will never exist again in all of human history. For a very short period of time, as the chromosomes sort themselves into the twenty-three pairs that each of this person's cells will now carry for the rest of his or her life, the person exists as a single cell called a zygote. Once that cell begins to divide, the process of human development proceeds at an astonishingly rapid pace. Barring illness or accidents of nature, the only thing that will now prevent the birth of this human being is the intentional intervention of abortion.

Within a very short period of only a few days, the new baby has begun to communicate with his or her mother. At this stage, the communication is via a biochemical message that is unmistakable to the mother's body. The new life within her begins to produce a hormone called *human chorionic gonadotropin.* This hormone, abbreviated as HCG, informs the mother's body of the new life within. This communication is vital. There is another hormone called progesterone. One of the mother's ovaries begins releasing progesterone at the moment of ovulation, even before conception, in order to prepare the uterus to host the new child that will result if conception occurs. Progesterone prepares the lining of the uterus to make it a hospitable place for the baby, and also helps to maintain a state of relaxation in the muscular wall of the uterus so that it will accommodate the growing child. If conception does not occur, then the ovarian production of progesterone ceases fourteen days after ovulation and the next menstrual period begins. Once the ovary detects the HCG being produced by the new baby, the production of progesterone will be maintained until the end of the first trimester. At that point, the placenta will be producing enough progesterone independent of the ovary, and the pregnancy will be maintained. It is at this point that the child has reached his or her first milestone of self-sufficiency.

The interaction between mother and baby is a delicate accomplishment. It only occurs because the child is a living organism, so much more than a "clump of cells." The mother's body begins to respond in many other ways because of this biochemical communication with her child. The way her body's insulin responds to her nutritional intake prepares the mother's body to store nutrients which will be needed in greater amounts as the baby grows. Her cardiac output begins to change, and her blood pressure and blood volume begin to change in ways that accommodate the growing baby. Her respiratory physiology begins to change in order to provide for the increased oxygen requirements—as you know, oxygen is vital to life. Since this child is alive, he or she needs oxygen. If the child was not alive, these accommodations would not be necessary. After all, toenails and tonsils don't change a woman's physiology. But if you listen to abortion advocates, they have compared the unborn child to those things exactly; and there is no shortage of other ludicrous metaphors they are willing to use to deny the life and humanity of the unborn.

All of these changes begin taking place in the first trimester, which ends at the gestational age of thirteen weeks from the beginning of the last menstrual period. During that incredibly busy time, much has happened for the child. During the fourth week after the last period, the baby's brain has become a distinct structure initially called the neural plate—just eighteen days after conception. Two days later, the brain and early spinal cord are visibly separate and distinct structures. Two days after that, just five weeks and one day after the last period and only three weeks after conception, the baby's heart begins to beat. Later that week, the earliest recognizable limbs are present as the arm and leg buds. During the early part of the next week, eyes, ears, a nose, and mouth are present. All these events are occurring during the embryonic period, which ends eight weeks after conception or ten weeks after the last menstrual period. This is when the child transitions from the embryonic stage of development to the fetal stage.

It is always amazing to me when those who support abortion say: "It's not a baby, it's a fetus." The word *fetus* is the Latin term for "little one," and is in no way an indication of the child's status as anything other than human. In like manner, the terms "infant," "toddler," "child," "adolescent," "teenager," and "adult" are not reflections of one being more or less human. These are simply terms which describe points along the timeline of the lifespan. As the child enters the fetal stage of development, he or she has ten fingers and ten toes—all of which have the same unique set of fingerprints, which will be carried throughout life.

Growth and development are rapid at this point. From the end of the fourth week to the end of the fifth week, the baby doubles in size. By the end of the embryonic period, he or she will have doubled in size two more times and will have all the structures needed for eventual life outside of the mother's body. All, then, that is needed is the passage of time to reach that point; and all this has happened before the end of the first trimester. The distinctions at different points during a pregnancy that have been drawn by the courts are completely arbitrary. Such distinctions are not grounded in scientific medical fact in any way, shape, or form.

The framework into which the Supreme Court, in 1973, placed the entire first trimester provides for the mother, in consultation with an abortionist, to be able to abort that pregnancy for any reason. *Roe v. Wade* prohibits the states from placing any restrictions whatsoever on abortion during that period of time. In doing so, the Supreme Court's seven justices, voting in the majority, concocted a line of reasoning never before employed in the history of legal jurisprudence. It not only denied that the unborn child is a person but also codified protections for those who seek to end the lives of unborn children.

While *Roe v. Wade* goes on to open the door for the individual states to enact some protections in a graduated way in the second, and then third trimesters, it does so in a completely arbitrary manner. You see, there is science and then there is social policy. The scientific facts which I have laid out for you are indisputable. They are a matter of unarguable scientific knowledge, proven over and again by extensive study and evaluation. These facts are taught to all medical students without exception. Science itself is neither right nor wrong, good nor bad, beneficial or harmful. Science is simply a sum total of knowledge and fact and has no innate goodness or evil.

Social policy is a matter of opinion. It is debatable and subject to changes of whim, and prone to wide swings based on shifts in political realities. Social policy can be good or can be evil. Social policy is always designed to provide some benefit for at least some members of society or for those in power. Social policy can be good, in that we have instituted social policies that protect children from abuse, that provide for a retirement benefit and for health care for our elderly, and that do any manner of other good things. Social policy can also be evil. Horrifically, slavery was an accepted social policy in the United States of America for almost a hundred years after the Declaration of Independence. Segregation in our schools, in the provision of health care, and in the arena of the service industry (among many others) was a widespread social policy for almost another hundred years. Nazi social policy enabled the murder of eleven million Jews, gypsies, homosexuals, and political dissidents. Communist social policy allows the mistreatment, imprisonment, torture, and murder of political opponents. Some countries have social policies that discriminate against those of a particular religious persuasion. All these social policies are evil, and they all have one key central tenet in common with the social policy of abortion: they dehumanize a particular class of human beings in order to make their mistreatment and/or their extermination more palatable to the remaining population, or to provide those in power with the ability to do so without obstruction.

Abortion dehumanizes the unborn child—a living, unique, individual human being. It says that the unborn child is completely disposable, simply because they are unwanted. Those who support abortion have chosen to deny the personhood of what science clearly shows is a human being. The position of science on the beginning of life and the human nature of the unborn is now so clearly known that it is, and always will be, a fixed point in time. The removal of personhood from that fact-based assessment of humanity was required for us to have today's current abortion policies in our country. Many fail to see the clear and present danger of our society having allowed this to happen.

While the scientific definition of life is fixed, the social policy of personhood is a floating point ungrounded in any reality other than current social whim. In 1973, when *Roe v. Wade* was decided, no one would have ever publicly advocated for killing a born-alive human being—either by active action or intentional neglect. In spring 2019, forty-four members of the Senate of the United States of America just advocated for that very thing.[7] Multiple states are now adopting legislation that would protect the practice of infanticide for children who survive an attempted abortion. The pro-abortion position was once that, "It's not a person worthy of protection until it is born and is alive," and now the position is, "It's only a person if it is born, is alive, and is wanted." This is the danger of divorcing subjective social policy from objective, provable reality.

Abortion is an institution which says that one person's "right" to a preferred lifestyle is more important than another person's right to life itself.

There is a reason that the "unalienable right to life" was the first liberty listed in the Declaration of Independence. It is the most important liberty, and when it is endangered for even one of us, it is endangered for all of us—because then we are all at risk of being on the wrong end of social policy. Such social policy is definitely not the type of moral principle held in high esteem by the Founders as they wrote the Constitution and the Bill of Rights, and is not the type of principle held in high esteem by a healthy society.

CHAPTER 2

ABORTION IS NOT HEALTH CARE

The efforts to advance abortion are relentless and increasingly aggressive. We have gone from Hillary Clinton in the 1990s, who said that abortion should be "safe, legal, and rare," to Hillary Clinton in 2018, who said we aren't doing *enough* abortions. Clinton wholeheartedly supported efforts by New York Governor Andrew Cuomo to codify radical new policies into New York law, as the state has now legalized abortion all the way up to the due date. Without exception, supporters of advancing abortion rights tell us that unlimited access to abortion services is a vital and crucial part of protecting women, empowering women, and providing important health care for women. There is even a current billboard campaign in my home state that posts an image of three smiling women with the message: "Abortion is health care and a human right." As with most other statements in support of abortion rights, this "message" is easily proven false if one only takes the time to examine the issue and the evidence.

Consider the regulation of legitimate health care. There is an entity called the Joint Commission that is responsible for the inspection and accreditation of more than twenty-one thousand health care organizations across the country. Its regulations carry the force of the law. The Joint Commission regulates all hospitals, free-standing ambulatory surgery centers, nursing homes, and other entities. Compliance with the Joint Commission is not optional. It is required for the maintenance of licensure everywhere, and for medical facilities to participate in Medicare and Medicaid. They have an inspection schedule with which every facility must comply. Some inspections are announced, and some are surprise visits. No facility has the right to turn a Joint Commission inspector away. The Joint Commission has a vast amount of authority. It will recognize those facilities that do things well and recommend necessary changes to facilities that need to improve. It has the authority to financially penalize and even close facilities that endanger patients. That is essentially the mission of the Joint Commission—to ensure the safety of patients in health care facilities.

The Joint Commission has standards which must be met for every single aspect of the care that patients receive. From floors to ceilings, physical structures in a medical facility must meet very high safety and cleanliness standards. Processes involving pharmaceutical drugs must be in place to reduce medication errors. Rigid infection control policies and processes for investigating and evaluating hospital-acquired infections must be in place and followed without exception. The proper function and maintenance of the hospital's sterilization processes, especially for surgical equipment, must meet all standards without exception. The tracking of outcomes for patients who suffer from infections is required.

Each and every person employed by the hospital must be able to demonstrate that they have been properly trained for what they do and are appropriately licensed and credentialed in the area of their responsibility—whether they are nurses, nursing aides, pharmacists, radiology technicians, surgical technicians, laboratory personnel, phlebotomists, physical therapists, speech therapists, or medical doctors. The provision of health care is perhaps the most highly regulated industry in our nation—with the least amount of forgiveness for errors and mistakes, and rightly so. All individuals working in hospital and in surgery center settings must be qualified to do that which they are employed to do. Because I am most familiar with the credentialing process for physicians, I will explain that to you in detail.

The credentialing process required for physicians in a hospital is almost as complex as the process to be granted top secret clearance. To be granted privileges at a hospital, the physician must complete an extensive application. Their entire education must be documented and verified. Their malpractice history, if any, must be carefully evaluated. Whether they have maintained continuing education programs is considered. Most hospitals require a physician to be board-certified, or at least be eligible to sit for the board examinations in their particular specialty and be making progress toward finishing that process. They must have good work references and character references. They must have a license to practice in the state in which they practice, and they must have a Drug Enforcement Agency certification that they are qualified to prescribe controlled substances. The physician's experience performing the procedures which he or she wishes to perform is placed under scrutiny.

Once a physician is properly credentialed and has been evaluated on all these measures by a committee of fellow physicians, privileges are granted only if it is found that the physician is qualified to care for patients in a safe and competent manner. This process is usually repeated every two years in a manner known as "recredentialing" to ensure that the physician continues to practice in a safe and effective manner. The process for a physician to obtain privileges at an ambulatory surgery center is almost as detailed—with one addition. Most surgery centers will require the physician be credentialed at and have admitting privileges to a nearby hospital facility. Only then can the physician transfer a patient who has had a complication during a procedure *to a hospital* for more definitive care services not available in free-standing surgery centers. One such common need is access to a blood bank, for patients with greater than expected blood loss.

The Joint Commission is not the only agency with which health care facilities must contend. Each state will have some sort of Department of Health that will have regulations with which compliance must be proven. Health Department inspectors inspect hospitals, surgery centers, and nursing homes to ensure the health and safety of those patients who use the facilities. They also inspect restaurants, barber shops, beauty parlors, nail salons, and tanning bed locations. Any place of business or any service industry location that provides food for the human body, or provides services that affect the human body, is subject to inspection. Every place, that is, except abortion clinics.

All this and I have yet to hardly scratch the surface of all that is in place to ensure patient safety. In the recent push for the Affordable Care Act, and for universal health care, the mantra from those who support those endeavors is that health care is a constitutional right. What you never see is a health care facility challenging these patient safety requirements on the basis that they are not necessary, too expensive, or are an undue burden on a patient's constitutional right to access health care. The health care industry complies because putting patient safety first is the right thing to do—and because they have no choice.

So why is abortion treated differently? Is it really different from legitimate health care, as I and those who agree with me insist? Or is it a respectable part of health care, one that is vital and necessary for women? And if so, why is it not regulated in the same manner that all other medicine is regulated?

The answer is this: the abortion industry refuses to be held to the same quality and safety standards that protect patients in all other fields of medicine. They care more about their bottom line; their disregard for the women they "serve" is cold, calloused, and financially motivated. They deflect, distract, and falsely claim that they are advocates for women. But they really only advocate for abortion—abortion without restriction, regulation, oversight, or accountability. Some may argue this is an overstatement. Let us evaluate the evidence.

Isn't knowledge power? Don't patients who are about to undergo a particular medical or surgical treatment deserve to know the details and risks? There is a process called informed consent. This is the process during which a doctor is expected to talk with a patient and explain the reasons for any procedure which has been proposed and considered, cover the alternatives, and clearly inform the patient of any complications which could be expected to occur. The patient must clearly understand the risks of possible adverse outcomes.

Planned Parenthood and other abortion rights groups have consistently opposed any laws which require clear and complete informed consent for abortion. If I do not clearly tell a patient about a complication which can occur during or after a surgical procedure, she can take me to court and sue me. Every month, I pay $3,500 to cover malpractice insurance, just in case something like that ever happens to me. If I were ever found to have a pattern of inadequate informed consent procedures, I could have my medical license taken away. When I discuss informed consent issues with a patient who is contemplating surgery, I inform them that—while I anticipate that their procedure will go well—there is always the possibility that complications could occur. When I am done with the discussion, they understand that they could develop a post-operative infection. They know that they could develop a post-operative deep venous thrombosis. I explain the measures we take to reduce the risk of these complications. They know that they could experience internal bleeding during or after surgery. They understand that other structures like the bladder or intestines could be damaged, and further surgery could be needed to repair such damage. They are also told that other serious or even fatal complications could occur.

In all cases of which I am aware, every state that has attempted to hold the abortion industry accountable to standard informed consent procedures has been challenged in court by the abortion industry in an effort to avoid the accountability that informed consent brings. Abortion advocates claim that they empower women. For one to truly empower an individual as they make an important decision, one must provide that individual with full and accurate information. When a provider fails to do so, then the patient may choose to proceed with a course of treatment that they would otherwise have declined.

States which have mandated an informed consent process that includes a waiting period have always been challenged as well. Waiting period laws have a clear rationale. The patient should hear all details about the proposed procedure and then have a brief period of time—in the case of abortion, most waiting periods are twenty-four to seventy-two hours long—in which they can consider what they have been told and decide if they really wish to proceed. Since an abortion, once performed, cannot be undone, why would anyone want such a decision to be made quickly or lightly?

There are already waiting periods required of women with regard to their reproductive health decisions. A permanent sterilization, also known to many as a "tubal," will permanently prevent pregnancy. A poor woman who relies on Medicaid for her health coverage and chooses to have a permanent sterilization will face a waiting period. The patient is required, by federal regulations regarding Medicaid, to complete an informed consent process, sign her consent form, and then wait a minimum of thirty days before having her sterilization procedure done. This requirement, that she wait a sufficient amount of time to be sure she wishes to make a permanent decision regarding her reproductive health, has never been challenged as an unconstitutional burden on her liberties. In fact, due to this federal regulation, I have seen countless women face some difficulties over the years. Let me explain. Poor women sometimes access prenatal care very late in the pregnancy. By the time they come for prenatal care and deliver at term, there hasn't been enough time for them to have signed the papers thirty days before they deliver. Thus, the woman cannot have their sterilization procedure at the time of delivery. Since they frequently do not come back for completion of post-partum care, often we do not see them again unless another pregnancy occurs.

If the woman delivers at term, past thirty-seven weeks, there are no exceptions to this rule. There is no consideration for the woman's late access to prenatal care. It is sometimes a burden upon women who cannot afford another child, and possibly already have several. The woman really did wish to have a permanent sterilization so that they would be finished with childbearing. Women's "advocates" have never challenged this thirty-day waiting period for sterilization, but they always challenge any waiting period mandated as part of the consent process for abortion. Apparently, it is fine to make them wait thirty days for a procedure that harms essentially no one. Yet abortion advocates find it unacceptable to wait even thirty minutes for a procedure that always ends the life of an innocent child.

What should a reasonable woman want to know about abortion and its potential complications in order to make an informed decision regarding the procedure? Here is a partial list[8] of complications:

- Abortion patients may develop post-abortive infection that will require additional treatment and which could result in chronic pain and loss of fertility.
- Abortion patients may have damage to the uterus and the cervix. The uterus can be perforated (punctured) during the procedure and other structures inside the abdomen can be damaged.
- Hemorrhaging may occur, resulting in significant blood loss.
- Abortion increases the risk of extremely premature delivery in future pregnancies, with the greatest additional risk seen in patients who have had three or more abortions.
- There is evidence that abortion may increase a woman's risk of future breast cancer.
- Post-abortive women are more likely to have drug and alcohol abuse problems.
- Abortion has been linked to an increase in mental health issues.
- A post-abortive woman is 2.6 times more likely to commit suicide.
- A post-abortive teenager is 10 times more likely to attempt suicide.
- As many as 52% of women who have undergone an early abortion and 67% of those who have undergone a late-term abortion will meet the criteria used by the American Psychiatric Association to diagnose post-traumatic stress disorder.

Abortion facilities do not want to have to tell women any of these things. They know that if they do, then fewer women will proceed with the process and pay them for doing so.

Another responsibility that any health care provider has when helping a patient decide on a treatment course it to discuss alternatives with the patient. In the case of abortion, the alternatives are obvious: the patient can choose to continue the pregnancy. Once delivery occurs, the woman can either parent that child or place the child for adoption. These are both legitimate alternatives. Did you know that, at any given point, there are approximately two million couples in America waiting to adopt a newborn?[9] Did you know that the average waiting time to adopt a newborn is somewhere between two and seven years? Given the rarity with which Planned Parenthood's clients choose these options, one must wonder how often such options are truly discussed.

There are other areas in which the abortion industry fights against the standards to which all of legitimate medicine is held. Earlier in this chapter, I explained the arduous process through which a physician must obtain admitting privileges. Some states have passed laws which require an abortion provider to have hospital admitting privileges at a nearby hospital, and those laws have been challenged. My home state of Tennessee currently has a law on the books which requires an abortionist to have admitting privileges at a hospital within the county in which the abortion is being performed or within an adjacent county.

Why is this important? Because complications occur during and after abortions. With any surgical procedure, when a complication occurs, the doctor most qualified to handle the complication will be the doctor who is most familiar with the procedure itself. Any doctor with an ounce of integrity will want to be able to provide the higher level of care needed when a patient experiences a complication. An abortionist whose patient experiences a complication can only provide that higher level of care when they can transfer the patient to a local hospital, meet them there, and provide the care for the complication. Reasonable people would think that this is simply a matter of common sense. But the abortion industry opposes such requirements and claims that it places an undue burden on the woman in her quest for an abortion. In actuality, it places a burden upon the abortionist that their powerful lobbyists find unacceptable—the burden of being able to provide quality care.

States which have attempted to place abortion clinics in the same category as ambulatory surgery centers have had their legislation universally opposed by the abortion industry. Abortion clinics will do many surgical abortions every year, and it is only logical to place them in the same class as other surgery centers… that is, if abortion is truly legitimate medicine like all other types of medicine, and if the lives and health of the women seeking abortion truly matter. Sadly, the courts have ruled that such requirements place an "undue burden" on the woman who seeks an abortion. Again, the true nature of the burden is on the abortionist.

The standards which must be met by surgery centers all pertain to patient safety, a fact which the abortion industry refuses to consider. They mock the requirement that hallways and doors be of a certain width. Yet they always fail to acknowledge that those requirements, when met, allow an emergency stretcher to be maneuvered into an operating room so that a patient with serious complications can be quickly and safely transferred from the operating table to a stretcher and out to an ambulance, to be taken to a hospital. Surgery centers with patient care on multiple floors are required to have elevators that can accommodate those stretchers, as it is not feasible to take a stretcher down a staircase.

Surgery centers also must demonstrate that the different personnel involved in patient care are properly trained and qualified to do the jobs to which they have been assigned. They must have proper infection control measures. Their autoclaves, the devices that sterilize surgical instruments, must be regularly tested to ensure that they are functioning properly. Patient infections must be reported to an infection control officer, who will evaluate what may have contributed to the infection and address the root cause. These are but two of the important requirements for which surgery center compliance ensures patient safety and the highest possible level of care. Abortion clinics have fought against these types of requirements at every turn.

These two specific examples are relevant to abortion clinics here in Tennessee. In the year 2000, Planned Parenthood sued the state of Tennessee and the state's Supreme Court "discovered" a fundamental right to abortion in our state constitution. After that, it was very difficult for the state legislature to pass any kind of meaningful regulation of abortion. Then, in 2001, one of our state's abortion clinic owners sued the state to block inspection requirements; he was victorious in court. Since then, the state health department could *ask* to be allowed to inspect an abortion clinic—but compliance was voluntary. When inspections were allowed, the health department would issue a report, but the clinics did not have to comply with the recommendations based on the findings.

Let's consider another industry as an example. When the health department inspects something as inconsequential as a nail salon and finds a problem, that salon will be given time to correct the deficiencies and then must submit to re-inspection. In the case of abortion clinics, those that *choose* to allow an inspection, compliance with the correction of deficiencies could not be enforced. In my research, I once downloaded the publicly available reports from the health department website on the five clinics which had chosen to allow an inspection. The reports of their deficiencies discovered ranged from nine pages to fifty-seven pages in length. Only one clinic allowed a re-inspection to demonstrate compliance—and its deficiencies were related to relatively trivial concerns, such as the posting of proper signage.

The other four clinics, with serious deficiencies, were unwilling to allow re-inspection to demonstrate that the issues had been corrected. The inspectors had documented deficiencies related to untrained personnel performing ultrasounds, the storage of patient medications in janitorial closets, and the improper prescription and dispensation of controlled substances. Most concerning, though, was that two of the five clinics had been notified by an outside agency, which monitors the test strips used in autoclaves to determine the sterility of the surgical instruments, that their autoclaves were not sterilizing the instruments. Notification had been provided to those two clinics in writing, by certified mail, and they had ignored these notices. They continued to use autoclaves which were not properly sterilizing the surgical instruments, and they did nothing to repair the autoclaves. These clinics did not allow subsequent inspections. All the women who had surgical procedures in these locations were at seriously increased risk of infection because the abortion clinics chose to prioritize cost over patient safety. Because the clinics also had no mechanism in place to track post-operative infections, as all legitimate health care facilities have, we will never know how many patients were harmed by the failure of these clinics to care about the women they served.

If abortion clinics were held to the same standards which legitimate medicine must respect, patients who seek abortion services would be at less risk for adverse outcomes and complications. These requirements would ensure that the people caring for women in need were properly trained for their responsibilities. They would require that medications were handled properly and that patients would not be exposed unnecessarily to potential infections. And if the abortion industry was primarily concerned with women's health, they would want to do everything possible to safeguard the women who seek their services. Since they oppose every effort to ensure patient safety, one can only conclude that the abortion industry cares more about the bottom line than about women.

We are always told that unrestricted access to abortion is a vital part of the complete health care package for women. Abortion advocates say that women with health problems will die by the thousands, or more, if they cannot access abortion services. They also claim that women died by the thousands before abortion was available in all fifty states. These statements, like so many of the so-called facts supporting abortion, are simply not true.

The very first baby I delivered would now be more than twenty-seven years old. I do not remember if that child was a boy or a girl. I do not remember the baby's name. What I do remember is the absolute sense of wonder in using my hands to usher a baby into the outside world and see that baby placed in the mother's arms. Since that time, it is reasonable to estimate that I have delivered somewhere in the neighborhood of seven thousand babies. I currently am in a solo practice and have built a database of over fourteen thousand active patients since establishing that practice thirteen years ago. In the years prior, I was in group practice settings in which the care of large numbers of prenatal patients was shared with other obstetricians—where I was involved in the prenatal care of far more patients than I actually delivered. It would be reasonable to estimate that I have been involved in the prenatal care of tens of thousands of women.

There are two very important statements of fact which I can make based on that experience. First, it is incredibly rare for a woman who is pregnant to have such a severe medical condition that ending an early pregnancy is required to protect and preserve her life. When such a problem is encountered before the point at which a living baby can be delivered and survive, and the woman is likely to lose her life if the pregnancy is continued to a point when the child can be delivered, then we have no choice. If the mother dies before the baby could survive if delivered, then both mother and baby die—which would be unacceptable. How often have I seen that? Twice. Two times only, out of all the pregnant women for whom I have cared in those twenty-seven years. Let's briefly review these two case examples.

The first case was a woman who had an unplanned pregnancy and was in her early forties. She had pulmonary hypertension and had a complex structural cardiac defect that included aortic stenosis. Her cardiologist was very concerned about her risk of mortality if she pursued continuing the pregnancy, as she had other medical co-morbidities that made the care for her conditions very complex. Upon being counseled regarding her options, she chose to terminate the pregnancy while still in the first trimester. After completing that, she returned to our clinic for a permanent sterilization procedure so that she would not have to face that choice again since she was not a good candidate for surgical repair of her cardiac issues.

The second patient was even more difficult. She was a young patient, in her early twenties, recently married and between twenty-one and twenty-two weeks along. She was transferred from her obstetrician in a community hospital in a rural part of the state, to the tertiary care center where I was training in Louisville, Kentucky. She had developed the most severe case of pre-eclampsia that I have ever seen. The woman was still more than two weeks away from being far enough along to expect the baby to survive if delivered. She was so ill that she most likely did not have two days to live, much less two weeks. She was in heart failure and her lungs were filling up with fluid. She was in kidney failure and liver failure, and her blood would no longer clot as her platelets were under 20,000 (normal is more than 150,000).

We had to choose between ending the pregnancy or watching her die along with her baby. We did the only thing we could. We used a powerful medicine to induce a rapid labor and within a few hours she delivered her baby. The child did not survive the delivery process and was stillborn—since both mother and baby were so ill. But the child was born intact, and she and her husband were able to hold their small child and grieve. The delivery began her recovery, and she was in the hospital for about a week before she had improved sufficiently to go home. She went on to have more children and did not have a recurrence of her blood pressure complication with the subsequent pregnancies. Abortion advocates would have you believe that these scenarios are common and that, without unrestricted access to abortion, thousands of women will die every year in the streets. This simply is not true. It generates sympathy for their case, but it is a false defense of abortion.

The second thing that my years of experience allow me to say concerns when a pregnancy is sufficiently advanced for the child to have a reasonable chance of survival if delivered. At that point, it is absolutely never necessary or beneficial to the mother for the pregnancy to be terminated by killing the child. Abortion advocates would have you believe that medical issues arise during the pregnancy that require it to end in order to safeguard the mother's life and health. They claim abortion saves women's lives and protects their health. Their first claim has some truth, while the second is absolutely false.

OB/GYNs, like myself, see women all the time who require an end to the pregnancy in order to safeguard their life and their health as they approach the end of the second trimester and during the third trimester. Women develop high blood pressure. Their diabetes becomes more difficult to manage. Perhaps they have lupus, arthritis, or epilepsy, and those conditions have worsened. They may have a problem with how the placenta is implanted, and they begin bleeding profusely. Events and conditions happen all the time that require us to deliver the baby and end the pregnancy to protect the mother. These events never require that the baby intentionally be killed as a part of the delivery process. The safest thing for the mother in these cases is also always the safest thing for the baby—achieve the delivery in the most safe and expeditious manner possible. This gives the mother the best potential outcome, and also safeguards the life of the child.

Abortion advocates have relentlessly tried to convince us all that the abortion process is faster and safer for the mother—and this is where the deception comes in. Abortion is not like the transporter on Star Trek that simply beams the baby out of the uterus and causes him or her to disappear quickly. Abortion kills the baby, whose corpse then must still be delivered from the mother's body. The difference between good obstetric health care and abortion is that good care makes the best effort possible to protect the baby. An OB/GYN delivers him or her in the fastest, safest way possible for the mother—while abortion requires extra steps before delivering the baby, in order to ensure that a dead baby's corpse is delivered instead of a living baby. The only purpose of late-term abortion is to ensure the delivery of a dead baby, a baby which still must be delivered, in order to "care" for the mother.

The extra maneuvers and procedures required to ensure the death of the baby before the delivery only add risk to the mother's process. If she is truly ill and needs to be delivered to safeguard her health, then anything that adds to her risk should be completely unacceptable to all involved. Modern obstetrics is good health care; late-term abortion is not health care at all. Late-term abortion is a social policy which permits risk to be added to the process of ending a pregnancy in order to achieve a social goal for the mother who does not want the child. The only true and real purpose of late-term abortion is to ensure that the baby is fully dead before he or she is fully delivered.

In regards to the claim that thousands of women died annually from illegal abortions prior to 1973, one need only look at data from the Centers for

Disease Control (CDC). The numbers regarding abortion deaths in America reported by the CDC show that, in 1972, the year before *Roe v. Wade*, there were only thirty-nine deaths in America from illegal abortion. That is a far cry from the claim of "thousands" of deaths due to illegal abortions each year. It is also important to remember that abortion was legal in a minority of states prior to *Roe*—and, in those states, twenty-four women died from legal abortions in 1972. Consider these figures carefully. Abortion was legal in certain circumstances in only twenty of the fifty states in 1972—yet almost as many women died from legal abortions in only twenty states, as there were who died from illegal abortions in all fifty states. The following year, in 1973, more women died from legal abortions than illegal ones.

These facts are certainly not consistent with the narrative that abortion supporters use on a regular basis. We now also know that there is no real way to know how many women are harmed or killed by abortion in America today. The abortion industry has fought all oversight, and many states do not require the reporting of abortion complications. Deaths related to abortion procedures are not consistently described as such on death certificates. Any numbers on abortion complications and mortality from any agency today will certainly be incomplete and inaccurate.

No matter how often they say it is, abortion is not health care. Pregnancy is not a disease, and abortion is not a cure. Abortion causes more problems than it solves. It is a permanent, irrevocable, and brutal solution to the temporary problem that unplanned pregnancy poses. Abortion is not a "freedom" and it is not a liberty. Any "liberty" that costs an innocent life each and every time it is exercised is not a liberty. It is a tyranny—of the powerful over the weak, of the loud and outspoken over the voiceless.

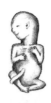

CHAPTER 3

WHEN ABORTION IS PART OF YOUR STORY

This chapter will include elements of full disclosure. Some of it will be simply practical, and much of it is painful.

The first disclosure is intended to proactively address something that could be used, in a way, out of context and twisted in order to discredit my words. My wife and I both worked at a Planned Parenthood location as part of our medical education in the mid 1990s. It is important to address this, and simply get it out there. Indeed, it is entirely in the realm of possibility that any Planned Parenthood effort to discredit the work of a pro-life individual would include, "Hey, this guy got paid by Planned Parenthood. Here is his W-2." Bear with me, and I will explain.

My wife, Julie, when we were dating, was working hard as a nurse in the busy Women's Pavilion of Norton Hospital in Louisville, Kentucky. At the time, it was by far the busiest obstetrics unit in the city. She covered shifts in Labor and Delivery, as well as on the Antepartum Unit for hospitalized high-risk patients whose medical issues required hospitalization for prolonged periods during the pregnancy. She was also an administrator and served as the Staff Educator for the Women's Pavilion. She was responsible for training and orientation of all nurses and staff in Labor and Delivery, the Antepartum Unit, the Post-Partum wards, and the Nursery. While doing this, and beginning to date me, she was also a busy single mother. Without getting into details, she had no choice but to divorce her first husband and had been divorced for approximately three years when we first met. Julie is an extremely bright woman with an incredible work ethic. While working full time and taking care of two precious children, a ten-year-old daughter and seven-year-old son, when we started dating, she was also in the Master's Degree in Nursing program at the University of Louisville. She was preparing to complete her training and sit for her Women's Health Nurse Practitioner certification exam. One of the required educational activities for the Master's in Nursing students who were pursuing certification in Women's Health was to spend clinical time at the Planned Parenthood location in the old part of downtown Louisville. It was an attractive building and had a fairly steady stream of clients. There were no surgical abortions done at that location; at that time, in the 1990s, medication abortion had not yet been approved in the United States. Patients came to this particular Planned Parenthood for Pap smears and birth control and minor gynecological problems. These were the patients that Julie saw and cared for. Any patients who came to that Planned Parenthood seeking abortion counseling or services were seen by a different nurse practitioner. That full-time Planned Parenthood employee was the only one who would be scheduled to see those patients, counsel them, and refer them to one of three different abortion providers functioning in Louisville at that time. Julie never saw a patient considering abortion in that clinic and was not paid for the time she spent seeing patients there.

Similarly, during the second year of residency training, all second-year residents had two months during which one of our responsibilities was to spend one afternoon a week seeing patients at Planned Parenthood. As with Julie's educational experience, our time was limited to seeing patients for Pap smears, birth control, evaluations of abnormal Pap tests, and minor problems of a gynecological nature. I never saw a patient with whom I had to even discuss abortion, as all of those patients were seen by the full-time Planned Parenthood staffer mentioned above. I was paid a small sum hourly for my time there, and that is why there may be a paper trail that says that I was once paid by Planned Parenthood. Understand, the rotation was not optional for those of us in our residency program. Because we were not involved in the abortion part of the institution, none of us could really object to being required to go. Abortions were not performed there, and we were not allowed to participate in seeing the patients who wished to obtain abortion services.

Understand that this is their pattern of practice. They wish to rigidly control the flow of information to clients who come to discuss an unplanned pregnancy. They would never have allowed an individual whose points of view might differ from theirs to discuss abortion with a vulnerable and scared client. I highly recommend the book written by Abby Johnson, *Unplanned*, in order that you might learn from a former insider how Planned Parenthood trains its people. We find they behave in ways worse than the worst used car salesman, to sell abortion to scared and vulnerable women. This book tells the story also dramatized in the recent movie by the same name.

As an aside, there is once again a push from those who support abortion rights, in both the government and medical education, to require those pursuing a career in obstetrics and gynecology to participate in abortion services. There have long been conscience considerations which allow individuals with an objection to abortion to decline to participate in such training, and one of the goals of the Obama administration was to systematically attack and disassemble those conscience protections. Sadly, the largest professional organization for obstetricians and gynecologists, the American College of Obstetrics and Gynecology (ACOG), has come into agreement with that agenda. ACOG has issued an opinion statement that an individual's personal beliefs as a provider of women's health should not be allowed to permit such an individual to decline training—nor, once fully trained and in practice, should they be allowed to decline to provide such services or refer for them. Fortunately, the Trump administration has taken steps to restore conscience protections before these abortion supporters make substantial progress toward such a wicked goal. That began as early as the mid 1990s, however. During the academic year 1995-1996, I served as the Chief Administrative Resident for the University of Louisville's Department of Obstetrics and Gynecology. That year, the Residency Review Committee, an accreditation entity responsible for regular review of accredited residency programs to ensure quality in training, issued a new requirement. It mandated that all accredited residency programs in OB/GYN offer training in the provision of abortion services to their residents. The new requirement did allow any resident that chose to opt out of such training to do so, but the decision to do so had to be given to the program director in writing. At that time, during my year as Chief, there were twenty-three residents in the program. All twenty-three signed the letter indicating their decision to decline such required training. There were, fortunately, no repercussions for any of us at that time. Some of us declined because we did not want to be trained to provide abortion services. Some, while being pro-choice, also did not wish to participate in such training because the physicians with whom we would have had to train were known for their questionable skills and practices. We had all seen or known about bad outcomes and could not bring ourselves to be involved in their abortion practices. I have digressed, but it is, perhaps, important to understand what was occurring in medical education at that time. It is also, now, very important that those responsible for educational policy be made to realize that they must never force anyone to participate in activities which they find personally unacceptable and objectionable.

Now, back to the full disclosure part. The painful part.

I am the father of a child who was aborted twenty-five years ago. I know from personal experience the almost incomprehensible pain, guilt, and shame that comes from a series of such bad choices. Both women and men for whom abortion is a part of their past can, and often do, suffer, usually silently.

There is no excuse and no rationalization sufficient for what we chose to do. Explanations, maybe. Justification? No. We tried to push it down and not think about it. That didn't work. We rarely talked about it and never disclosed it to anyone else. That did not make it go away. We knew that God forgives, and that at the moment of salvation all sin—past, present, and future—is forgiven. But even that head knowledge didn't heal the heart, and it didn't fill the holes in our hearts. It didn't answer a single one of the many "what if's?" And there were so many of those "what if's?"

We both would have called ourselves pro-life at that time, but we were by no means activists on the issue. We had never been in prayer outside an abortion clinic. We had taken no public stand on the issue. And while we both found the practice of abortion concerning and distasteful, we had devoted no significant time or thought to the issue. We were both so busy, so stressed, and so in love that we rationalized away our choice to be intimate before we were married. Then, it happened. We were pregnant. Julie was so busy working, raising two children, and trying to finish her master's degree. I was working so hard as a resident in my final year with so many responsibilities. We had plans to marry, move, and start a new season in our lives. We told ourselves that we just couldn't do everything that we had to do. We told ourselves that we didn't want to set a bad example for the two children we knew we would be raising together. Honestly, we didn't want to deal with the embarrassment of an unplanned pregnancy at such an inconvenient time. We didn't want to disappoint our families.

That, you see, is the problem with sin. It draws you in and works to reduce your discomfort with it. It gives you the rationalizations needed to get you farther down the road than you ever thought you would go. You then reach a point when it is too late. What would have been unthinkable to us became less and less unthinkable. It began to seem like the least difficult option. How wrong we were.

I will tell you why I feel that I bear the largest responsibility for our mistake. It was not the first mistake. I have come to realize that the genesis of this set of mistakes is found in what my priorities were at the time. Medical school and residency are intensely busy, with unyielding demands on time. I had fallen out of regular worship attendance. Daily devotional time did not happen. My prayer life was almost nonexistent. When faced with the most difficult personal situation I had encountered up to that point, I lacked the strength that would have come from a closer walk with my Creator. Had I been the man God created me to be at that time, we probably wouldn't have been in that situation anyway; even if we had, it would have been handled differently. Is that a justification? Absolutely not. It is a simple fact. Tragic and heartbreaking certainly, and still inexcusable in my mind.

Post-abortive people struggle with depression, self-loathing, and anger. There can be other manifestations, but those were ours. We manifested our struggles differently, as you might assume men and women would. I became intensely angry at the abortion industry and the hands who profited from taking innocent lives. Julie, on the other hand, turned her anger inward and struggled with more severe bouts of depression. Both of us struggled under the weight of self-loathing and spent many years trying to work hard to feel good about ourselves. We both stuffed our experiences. It would take two decades before we actually even brought it up to each other in meaningful conversation. Not healthy, I know—but also probably not that uncommon for our generation.

For most of this time, I worked actively as a pro-life activist. But I have come to learn that this does not mean that I adequately dealt with my own pain and emotions from being post-abortive. It was easy to fuel my passion with anger rather than to do the necessary work that it really takes to heal. It took me too long to understand the difference and, quite honestly, to accept my own actions and the consequences of them.

Things reached a crescendo for Julie and I. Ultimately, the pain became too great to bear. I genuinely believe that God orchestrated this time for both of us so that we could really begin to do the necessary work that is required. Part of healing is acknowledging the truth of the damage that was incurred. Then one begins to appropriately work through the grieving process of that loss. Julie started first working with a Christian counselor. She did the Surrendering the Secret Bible study on her own and then in a group setting. Now, she has done the leadership training for that study and has begun facilitating this study for other post-abortive women. Healing was not an instantaneous occurrence. Yet she was the most surprised at how much God showed up for her during such a sorrowful and broken season of her life. He was faithful, despite our brokenness and sin.

My journey has been different. I had tried so hard to atone for what I had done. I came to realize that there are simply some things for which atonement on our own cannot be accomplished. It is only by appropriating what Christ did for us and for all of our sin that we can deal with the things that we have done.

One resource that has helped me see things more clearly has been a book titled *Healing a Father's Heart*, by Linda Cochran and Kathy Jones. Both of them had experience helping post-abortive women. They decided to assemble a post-abortive strategy for men, when they realized that men had no specific resources available to them and were using books designed with women in mind.

In their well-designed book, the most important chapter for me personally was the chapter on anger—which had been my predominant reaction to the reality of what we had done. That, and denial. In one chapter, they discuss how relief and denial are the two most common immediate reactions that men have once an abortion has been done. Some men are immediately relieved, as they had thought that having to be a father before being ready was the worst problem they had ever faced. I cannot say that relief is something I felt. I felt loss and went into denial... and that suppression of reality led to anger and all the problems that being chronically angry brings.

So often, the choice to proceed with an abortion goes against everything we think we are and what we think of ourselves. This leaves us with a dichotomy that is irreconcilable on our own. For me, specifically, I chose obstetrics and gynecology because by nature I am a fixer and I want to be happy. Early in medical school, I realized that I would not have done well with chronic disease management instead of cures. I wanted to be a part of the exciting times that having a baby brings to families. Additionally, most problems one will encounter as an OB/GYN have either a medical or a surgical solution, and are, thus, "fixable." Abortion promises to "fix" the problem of the unintended, inconvenient, or unwanted pregnancy. Men want to fix things. We want solutions. With abortion, one quickly discovers that abortion doesn't "fix" anything; it is not a "solution" to anything. Abortion is a bigger problem than the unplanned pregnancy, and it only makes things worse for everyone involved. I quickly came to painfully know that we had fixed nothing. What we had chosen was not a solution in any sense of the word. Then, denial led to decades of pain and dysfunction.

When abortion is part of your story, whether you are a man or a woman, don't fall into the traps of guilt, shame, embarrassment, anger, bitterness, and resentment. These are all dark and damaging emotions, and the solution is to bring light into the situation. Deception is all dark and shadowy, but truth brings light and life. Be open with each other, if you are still together, about what happened and how you feel about it. Seek professional counseling if you need help in beginning to know how to deal with such strong and powerful feelings. Study books and programs like *Surrendering the Secret* and *Healing a Father's Heart* can be so very helpful. If your church has a strong post-abortive component in its overall ministry program, then take advantage of that. Lastly, consider your local crisis pregnancy centers, as many of them will offer post-abortive counseling.

Finally, once you feel that you are solidly on the path to being healed and once again whole, consider being a part of helping others heal. Be a part of sidewalk ministry or volunteer at a pregnancy center to help others avoid the same mistake. Educate yourself on the topic and be able to discuss it with others. Become a voice for the voiceless. Be the salt and light we are commanded to be. If you are so inclined, begin to participate in the political and legislative process and make those in politics aware of the fact that you will be watching what they do on the issue of life and you will vote accordingly. We cannot directly affect judicial decisions, but we can affect the legislative process. Politicians respond to pressure and to money. Donate to truly pro-life candidates if you are able. Most definitely, vote against those who are pro-choice or those for whom being "pro-life" is little more than a bullet point on a campaign poster.

I will offer you one bit of advice, learned from personal experience. Do not rely on activism to bring your healing. Allow your feelings to motivate your actions, but don't equate success in activism to healing. It simply will not work.

If we are to see a change in our society on the issue of abortion, we must approach it in three different ways. One is truthfully making people aware of its ugly reality. Deception is how the other side has made the progress it has. Once the knowledge of the reality of abortion becomes more prevalent, abortion itself becomes more unthinkable. Another is to be truly caring for the woman who needs help through a pregnancy. She must see that there are options other than ending the pregnancy, and those options must be realistic. Ending abortion on demand will not solve the issues faced by those who have an unintended pregnancy, and we must take this under consideration as part of the strategy. The third way is to continue to hammer away at it legislatively and politically.

The one thing that will not work, in your personal life or in the public arena, is continued silence. Silence enables abortion to flourish. Silence gives it power. Raising your voice takes that power away.

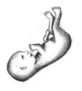

CHAPTER 4

REFUTING ABORTION'S RATIONALE

*"And yes, words matter. They may reflect reality, but they also
have the power to change reality – the power to uplift and to abase."*
William Raspberry

William Raspberry was a Pulitzer Prize-winning columnist who wrote more than five thousand columns and was published in over two hundred newspapers in his almost forty years as a writer. His commentary above on the power of words is important, appropriate, and relevant to this topic. Words do matter, and they really can change reality. In the case of abortion, the words chosen by those who support abortion really have changed reality.

Prior to 1973, abortion was unthinkable to most people. That changed because of the words chosen carefully and used repeatedly by abortion supporters. It was not some new scientific discovery or medical advance that caused the unborn child to be dehumanized. The perceived status of the unborn child changed because the supporters of abortion labored to convince people that the child was no more than a clump of cells, or a blob of tissue, or a clot of blood. How unborn babies were perceived and treated began to shift as women were portrayed as victims and the nature of life in the womb was ignored. The issue was framed as one in which the right of the woman to terminate a pregnancy was pitted against the right of the state to regulate abortion—and *the right of the child to live* was ignored. Abortion began to be thought of as a social good. Once we as a nation were on that slippery slope, the abortion industry relentlessly pursued an agenda in which abortion rights are ever expanding.

Nothing is allowed to stand in the way of abortion without restriction, without regulation, without oversight or medical quality assurances. They permit no discussion of the child or tolerance for those who are convinced of the humanity of the child. America is now one of only seven nations on the planet that allow abortion after twenty weeks; other nations in this notorious club include such bastions of human rights as China and North Korea. Is this where we want to be as a society? Did the Founders envision, as they penned the Constitution and the Bill of Rights, a time when we would have to argue that killing our children should not be a liberty protected by due process and rights to privacy?

In this battle, wins and losses are decided because of the strength of the words used. Judicial opinions are words on paper crafted together in response to arguments consisting of words presented to the courts. Legislative actions ultimately are words on paper assembled by the legislators, whose opinions prevail during debates and discussions in Congress and in state houses all over America. Words matter. Words convince people. Words changed the reality of how the child is perceived and treated. And convincing words are the only way we will be able to turn the tide and restore any semblance of humanity to the unborn child and how he or she is treated. Legislators must be convinced, judges must be convinced, and, most importantly, the people must be convinced. This will only occur when enough of us know the truth and are equipped to speak the truth, using words to counter that which is spoken by those anti-life, pro-abortion forces. If we are to change the reality of abortion in America, we must be able to use words truthfully and to our advantage.

Defenses of abortion usually fall into one of a small number of justifications. These are relatively easily overcome with a basic understanding of the issues. Before I dive into these, I will recommend two other books for anyone who wishes to pursue a far more thorough engagement with pro-life apologetics. *Pro-Life Answers To Pro-choice Arguments* by Randy Alcorn[10] is excellent, as is *The Case for Life* by Scott Klusendorf[11].

The primary tactic used by those who support abortion on demand without restriction is to convince the listener that the baby in the womb is not really a human. Statements along those lines go something like this: "It's not a baby, it's a fetus." Or, "It's just a clump of cells, blob of tissue, clot of blood." Or, "Having an abortion is no different than having a tonsillectomy." This tactic of dehumanizing a class of people you then wish to mistreat is common throughout history. African Americans were not thought of as being fully people due to their skin tone, and that belief was used to justify owning them as slaves. Jews were said to not be human at many points in history, and that belief was then used to justify the Holocaust. Women were not thought of as being equal to men and were denied the right to vote— even here in America, until just one hundred years ago. Even now, women are not thought of as fully people in many places in the world.

While these beliefs are no longer tolerated in America, there are those who sincerely have no moral qualms about abortion because they believe the lie that the child in the womb is not yet a person. That belief, as discussed in the first chapter of this book, is clearly refuted by an understanding of science and medicine which demonstrate that life begins at conception. When challenged by anyone on this issue, or told by anyone that medical science does not tell us when life begins, point to those examples I cited. Then ask your fellow conversant to point to one single, peer-reviewed medical or scientific journal article or scholarly textbook actually used in scientific or medical education that says that science does not know when life begins. They will be able to quote none—not one single source.

"You can't force your religion on me." "Stop trying to legislate morality." "This is none of your business." Each and every one of these rather silly statements can also be simply refuted. While I am a person of faith, and my faith shapes how I interact with the world around me, I do not have to use my faith to defend the pro-life point of view. Science proves the point that human life begins at conception. Civilized society in every other situation demands that the strong protect the weak, that the powerful defend the defenseless, and that those who can speak have an obligation to speak for the voiceless. That is civil, moral, and right. In order to argue against these points, one must be willing to discriminate against the weak, the defenseless, and the voiceless. Tell your opponent that you can defend the pro-life point of view without mentioning your faith, and then do so. This completely defuses the "faith" objection to the pro-life point of view. They will then, typically, turn to the even weaker arguments that you cannot legislate morality and that it is none of your business. There are also straightforward responses to these arguments.

All law is legislated morality. Each and every law that regulates human behavior is the legislative enactment of what some group of legislative individuals has decided is moral, correct, and right. We have decided that it is wrong to murder another human, wrong to sexually assault an individual, and wrong to steal. Laws uphold the standards that it is wrong to beat your wife or your child, and it is wrong to drive at eighty miles per hour through a school zone—especially when the school zone lights are flashing. There are literally hundreds of examples of things which civilized society has decided are immoral behaviors. Why? Because they can result in harm to others. Civilized society has thus enacted rules and laws against such behaviors. To say that "you cannot legislate morality" is simply nonsensical.

Along similar lines, when someone says "it is none of your business" we must ask them this: If you pull into your driveway and you see your next-door neighbor beating his three-year-old child with a baseball bat, is that any of your business? Do you call 911? Do you run to the child's defense? Do you try to stop the atrocity from happening? Or do you simply park your car, check your mail, and wander on into your house and start dinner... because you believe you have no basis to defend the defenseless child from certain severe injury or death? This argument, in an effort to silence those who hold deep convictions about the humanity of the unborn, is an argument that a pro-abortion person would find very unpopular if they used it to try to defend the child abuser. Yet far too many in the pro-life community find themselves woefully unprepared to speak forcefully and with conviction when confronted with statements that are simply wicked.

You see, these points are all sound bites. They are easy to remember and repeat as if you are no more than a parrot. Many of the people who will challenge a pro-life person do not even realize that they are parroting sound bites that have no basis in science, logic, reason, or fact. These statements simply sound good to them, so they eagerly repeat them.

Now let us tackle one that is a bit more complicated. That is not to say that it is difficult to combat, but it does require a bit more savvy to refute. It is the "my body, my choice" argument. This point of contention, this justification for ending the life of the unborn child, is that the child resides within the body of another person. Ethicists call this the bodily autonomy argument. It essentially says that no one has the right to control what one does or does not do with his or her own body, and that demands on one's body against their will cannot be made. This line of logic says that the right to make decisions about one's own body reigns supreme over all other considerations. Those who use this argument will sometimes draw the analogy that one cannot be compelled to donate blood or an organ, even though another person who happens to need it may die without it. U.S. law does not even allow organs to be taken against one's will after they have died, even though such action may save others. They draw an inappropriate equivalence between these situations and pregnancy, and claim that the unborn child is making a demand of the woman's body that the woman has the right to refuse.

This point of contention can be addressed on multiple levels. One must understand that bodily autonomy does not reign supreme as a right in medicine, or in the law. We do not allow those under eighteen to purchase tobacco products, even for their own personal use. We do not allow those under eighteen to get tattoos. We do not allow those under twenty-one to purchase or consume alcohol. And all those restrictions are the result of our having decided that protecting one from certain choices is a social good, because without those protections someone may bring harm to themselves and even to others. Abortion, as I have discussed in earlier parts of this book, sometimes does bring harm to the woman; and it *always* brings death to someone else. The body destroyed by someone who pursues abortion based on the "my body, my choice" argument is not their own body, but is the body of another unique living human being who happens to temporarily reside inside of the pregnant individual.

There are other situations in medicine in which bodily autonomy is not allowed to dictate that we allow self-harm, or that we allow someone to be harmed by another. As a medical professional, I am required to be a mandatory reporter. That obligation says that when I see a woman in my office who is being beaten by her husband, I am required to report the situation if it has not already been addressed by law enforcement or social services. The woman may object, and may say that she doesn't want me to report it because she has a right to choose to stay with him no matter what he does. Since he isn't beating anyone else, is it anyone one else's business? That position and opinion on her part does not free me from my legal and ethical obligations.

If I see a patient who is suicidal, I am obligated to involve mental health professionals and, if necessary, sign commitment papers which take away all bodily and individual autonomy in order to commit the patient to a mental health facility in which she can be evaluated. She will not be released from such a facility until the professionals caring for her have deemed that she is no longer a danger to herself. It is her body, but she does not have the right to take active action to destroy that body. If she has voiced intent to harm another, I am also obligated to report and participate in detaining her. In the same vein, we also have decided as a society that it is sometimes permissible to commit a minor patient with disorders like anorexia to a facility in which she can be treated, and force fed if need be, with no regard for her "bodily autonomy." The minor child who is engaged in self-mutilation can be compelled to undergo evaluation and treatment. The bodily autonomy argument does not allow us to overlook situations in which harm is brought to self, or to another individual, based on the bodily autonomy point of view.

Then we hear the argument: "It is a woman's private decision, between her and her doctor, and no one has the right to interfere." Sometimes it's between only her and her family, or her clergyman. In *Roe v. Wade*, the Supreme Court ruled that a woman had a right to privacy under the Due Process Clause of the Fourteenth Amendment. The Court's ruling says that a right to privacy contained in the Fourteenth Amendment covers the choice to have an abortion. Privacy sounds like an appealing thing, doesn't it? Who wants to argue against anyone's privacy? In the world of medicine, privacy is especially prized. Patients expect to have their privacy maintained, and current HIPAA laws impose severe penalties on health care facilities and individuals who inappropriately disclose confidential information or breech a patient's privacy. This right to medical privacy, however, is not without exception.

When a patient is diagnosed with certain sexually transmitted infections—like gonorrhea, syphilis, or chlamydia—then the law requires that a report be made to the health department. The health department will then assess, based on an interview with the patient, any need for partner notification and evaluation and treatment. Privacy laws and regulations find themselves secondary to the need to prevent harm to another.

Let us consider another scenario. Suppose I enter an exam room to see a patient who has come to me for help, because she is convinced her life is in danger. She has a black eye, a busted lip, a missing tooth, and has bruises and scrapes on her arms. I ask her what happened to her, and she confides in me that her husband comes home from work each evening, drinks a fifth of whiskey, and demands dinner. If he is not pleased with the quality of the food, he beats her. The beatings have been increasing in frequency and severity. She has not reported this because she fears him. Last night, he beat her more badly than ever before—and told her that the next time he didn't like the food, he would kill her and find another wife. She is entirely convinced that she will soon die if the situation does not change. She then calmly, rationally, and thoughtfully asks me for a prescription for a barbiturate sedative that she knows she can add to his bottle of whiskey. She knows that if he drinks that when he gets home, he will lose consciousness, stop breathing, and die. Then her life will no longer be in danger.

Does her right to privacy allow me to honor her request to take active action to bring harm to another individual even though it will save her life? No, it most certainly does not. Her right to privacy does not enable me to take action to end someone else's life, even though the reprehensible actions of that individual endanger her life. Her right to privacy also does not allow me to keep her situation confidential, even though she begs me to do so. She pleads insistently that I not notify the authorities because she fears that the danger to her life will increase. Her right to privacy and her fear for her life do not allow me the discretion to decide not to report. I am a mandatory reporter and required to involve law enforcement and/or social services, so that she can obtain help and protection properly. Her life truly is in danger. Even given that fact, her right to privacy does not entitle her to take active action to bring harm, as deserved as it may be, to another individual.

Yet this is exactly what happens when a woman, in consultation with her doctor, makes a "private" decision to end the life of an unborn child. Private or not, abortion is a decision to bring ultimate harm to a completely innocent and helpless individual. Privacy laws and constitutional protections are used to justify abortion in ways that are never used in application to any other situation in the law or medicine.

Then they say, "If you don't have a uterus, you don't have a say"—wishing to silence all male critics of the institution of abortion. In an excellent article[12] published in *The Federalist*, Care Net President and CEO Roland C. Warren addresses this issue. He correctly points out that this argument is no more than a sound bite, and contains no sound logic. In fact, if all male input on abortion is to be disregarded, then we should start by sending *Roe v. Wade* to the trash can—as it was decided by seven of the nine members of the Supreme Court of the United States before the first female justice was appointed. All nine members were men, and eight of the nine were white.

In a time when the Left is tired of hearing from "old white men," they sure do want to cling to that supremely wrong piece of jurisprudence decided by a bunch of elderly and mostly white men. This insistence on a form of leftist-approved sexism is easily shown to be hypocritical.

As Warren points out in the article, there are a number of examples of times when supporters of abortion have sought to enlist men to be "bro-choice" and to be supporters of abortion rights. The leftist pro-choice treatment of pro-life men is much like the leftist treatment of conservative blacks. It is disdainful, disrespectful, demeaning, dismissive, and hypocritical. They try to distract you and deflect pro-life arguments that are voiced by men, just as they try to silence conservative blacks. Rachel Maddow has famously said, "If you don't have a vagina, you don't get to make laws regulating them." The problem with Ms. Maddow's position is that regulating abortion is not the same as regulating someone's vagina. Such a position is completely ludicrous. By Maddow's standard, men should not pass laws against prostitution or sex trafficking either. Here is a simple truth. The purpose of any anti-abortion law is not to regulate anyone's vagina. The purpose is to prevent the killing of an innocent unborn child, whether that killing is done by a procedure that enters the uterus through the vagina or done by administering medication without entering the vagina at all. Leftist defenders of abortion have a way of trying to reduce the argument to vulgar sound bites that are not based on reality or truth in any way. Such arguments are completely devoid of common sense and are relatively easy to refute if you just give the issue some thought.

Another similar argument is that pro-life people should stay "out of other people's bedrooms." The premise is that we have no business being involved in what happens in the privacy of someone's bedroom. Rest assured, no pro-life advocate wants to enter other people's bedrooms. The problem the supporter of abortion rights has with this argument is this: abortions aren't performed in bedrooms. Abortions are performed in clinics or by medications administered in clinics and are not occurring in the private bedrooms of the private homes of the individuals who conceived the unplanned child. Another piece of the hypocritical puzzle we see here is that while the abortion rights supporter demands that the pro-life individual stay out of their bedroom, they also demand that we contribute to the financial cost of contraception and abortion. We aren't allowed to have a say, but we have to pay so they can play. This position is simply and indefensibly ludicrous, and it is easy to call it out for what it is.

Another set of arguments that you will encounter is that abortion is necessary because of poverty. Supporters of abortion will argue that unfettered access to abortion is necessary to reduce the poverty experienced by women, and that it is an injustice to allow children to be born into impoverished families. Facts, however, are wonderful things. If abortion is really necessary to reduce poverty, then we should see a reduction in poverty rates since the advent of abortion in all fifty states after *Roe v. Wade*.

Using Census data, we can look at poverty rates in 1973, when *Roe* was decided, and compare them to poverty rates now. Supposedly, abortion helps impoverished women and reduces the number of children who grow up in poverty. Thus, we should see definite drops in the poverty rates in those groups. Yet, that is not what a careful examination of the data shows. In 1973, the number of women ages 18-64 living at or below the poverty line was 10 percent. In 2016, forty-three years after *Roe*, the number of women ages 18-64 living at or below the poverty line is 13.4 percent. That is not a drop that corresponds with widely available abortion—it is an increase.

In 1973, 14.9 percent of children under age eighteen lived in homes with a single female head of the household. In 2016, that number was 24.9

percent. Abortion didn't reduce the number of children living in households headed by a single female. It also did not reduce the poverty rate of those children. In 1973, 54.7 percent of children under age eighteen living in a home headed by a single female lived at or below the poverty line. In 2016 that number was 59.5 percent.

Abortion supporters point to a study published in March 2018. *The American Journal of Public Health* released a research article[13] titled "Socioeconomic Outcomes of Women Who Receive and Women Who Are Denied Wanted Abortions in the United States." Some of the authors are faculty members of the University of California, San Francisco and one is a part of Ibis Reproductive Health, an abortion advocacy group in Oakland, California. Their study design allowed them to conclude that women who were denied a desired abortion are indeed more likely to experience poverty. It ostensibly focused on a woman who wants an abortion but is unable to obtain one. They say she is more likely to experience long-lasting poverty.

Their study design looked at the socioeconomic status of women seeking abortions at any of thirty different abortion centers between 2008 and 2010. They looked at women who presented for an abortion just before the cutoff age at their particular abortion center and were able to obtain the abortion. They compared their socioeconomic status later to the status of women who presented just after the gestational age cutoff at the particular center and were unable to obtain the abortion. They concluded that there are significant adverse differences in the group who was turned away from having a desired abortion when compared to the group able to obtain their desired abortion.

The study fails to acknowledge several confounding factors clear in the data. First, it mentions significant differences in demographics of the groups at baseline. But it fails to acknowledge that these differences could be responsible for the increased poverty seen over the subsequent five years. Women who were unable to obtain the abortion were far more likely to be under the age of twenty and unemployed at the time they sought the abortion. They were also more likely during the five years of follow-up to have been raising children alone, with no partner or meaningful assistance from the fathers of the babies. The only explanation is that the authors desired to focus on denial of abortion services as the root cause of poverty. They refused to consider how the failure of the family unit has contributed to the impoverishment of young women with children.

Of course, it draws fiery criticism to say that men should be involved in the lives of the women with whom they father children. It draws criticism to say children with absentee fathers are more likely to be impoverished. It will be said that drawing such conclusions is sexist—but it is reality.

The census data is clear. Poverty rates for women went up after *Roe v. Wade*. Specifically, poverty rates for children living in single parent homes led by a woman rose significantly after that infamous decision.

What caused these changes is likely multi-factorial. It may have more to do with the failure of the family unit than with whether abortion is easily available. One conclusion we can certainly draw from this data is that the increased abortion access after *Roe* certainly did not reduce poverty rates for women or their children. The current mainstream insistence that laws which limit abortion access will increase poverty is nothing more than disingenuous hysteria. It is intended to sway public opinion and distract from the facts. These laws are not intended to be punitive to women but, instead, are an outflow of the conviction that all life is worthy of protection.

We are intended to believe that abortion supporters are really advocates for women, especially for women who struggle with poverty or women in minority groups. I will share with you one story of how the abortion industry does not care about impoverished women.

In my career as an obstetrician, I have not only delivered thousands of babies; I have also been involved in the care of many more thousands whom I ultimately did not deliver. One African American woman whom I encountered several years ago, I will never forget. Poverty required her to be on Medicaid for her health care, as she had no other options. At the end of the first trimester, an ultrasound exam diagnosed her baby with a universally lethal condition known as acrania—the condition in which there is a brain but there is no skull. This is rare, and is always lethal. The diagnosis was confirmed by the specialist to whom we referred her for a second opinion. She was appropriately counseled on the situation by me and by the specialist she saw. She was truthfully told that carrying the child to term and delivering did elevate her risk of complications during delivery. It increased her risk of needing a Cesarean section, even though her other babies had been born naturally. This also would add to her risk, as she was obese and had other medical co-morbidities.

She asked the specialist and me whether abortion was an option. The specialist told her it was, and she asked what I thought. I told her that adding to her own risk when she had other children to care for was something she would have to consider carefully. If she chose to proceed with an abortion, we would help her afterward with any needs she had. And if she chose to carry, I said I would take care of her. She was leaning towards abortion, and she scheduled an appointment with one of Nashville's abortion providers. At that time, one was Planned Parenthood and the other was owned independently by a gynecologist who operated two facilities in Tennessee. She never told me which facility she went to visit.

Now, understand that Medicaid will pay for pregnancy termination when it is medically indicated. She went to her appointment with the documentation from the specialist who confirmed the child's diagnosis and its lethality. You must also understand that when a medical provider has a contract with Medicaid, they must accept Medicaid reimbursement for covered procedures. It is a violation of federal law to refuse to accept that amount and instead demand payment from the patient. Both facilities had contracts with Medicaid because they saw Medicaid patients for annual exams and birth control.

Medicaid will pay somewhere in the neighborhood of two or three hundred dollars for a late first trimester or early second trimester abortion. The cash price at the facility to which she went was $800. The facility refused to accept Medicaid reimbursement for the procedure, a violation of federal law. They did not care about the poor, pregnant woman whose child had a lethal anomaly and who had other children for which she needed to care. They didn't care about her sadness, poverty, or brokenness. They only cared about the cash, even though such an action violated what was legal and ethical.

The abortion industry doesn't care about poor women. It only cares about cash. Their insistence on discussing abortion in the context of poverty is simply a ploy to create sympathy for a "victim" group in order to protect their cash cow. Incidentally, my patient did not have $800, so she had no choice but to continue the pregnancy. She came to the office for an appointment at nineteen weeks. We discovered that the child had already died in utero. I then scheduled her for a labor induction and we delivered her non-living child intact. She was able to mourn and then move on. In this case, as in many others, the pro-life doctor took care of the woman with a sad and tragic situation. Meanwhile, the abortion industry slammed its door in her face.

Then there are those who demand that abortion is necessary to protect women from having to deliver children that are known to have disabilities, defects, or diseases. Ultrasound technology has allowed us to predict with a great degree of specificity (but not infallibility) the presence or absence of defects, and blood tests now exist that predict (also not perfectly) a patient's risk of having a child with Down's syndrome or other similar conditions. Laws have been passed in some state houses that would make it a violation of the law to perform an abortion because the child is thought to have Down's syndrome. Such laws are always challenged by the abortion industry, because they want to continue to be able to abort as many pregnancies as possible. For them, any excuse is a good excuse to make a buck.

One problem with this mindset should be obvious to any rational and reasonable person. We as a nation care about people with disabilities. The Individuals With Disabilities Education Act was passed in 1973, the same year as *Roe*. We care about children with disabilities and have rightly passed legislation which provides for accommodations in public education for those children with varying levels of ability. In fact, in higher education programs today, students who are interested in serving and educating those children are encouraged to think of them as "children with varying levels of ability" instead of "disabled" or "handicapped" children. This view allows us to focus on what an individual can accomplish instead of what they cannot do. The abortion industry and its advocates do not see children with varying levels of ability—they see a reason to profit from the eradication of anyone whose level of potential function fails to rise to some arbitrary standard. They promote this as a somehow compassionate view—as if brutally killing someone based on their level of ability is appropriate. Holding such disparate views in our society renders the foundation of all our human rights unstable. Consistency in how we view life and personhood and humanity brings stability and allows us to address issues fairly.

After the legislation mandating provisions for the education of those with varying levels of ability, the Americans With Disabilities Act was enacted. This piece of legislation recognizes the rights of those with varying levels of ability to participate as fully as possible in society. It makes it illegal to discriminate against any individual on the basis of any disability that they might have. Not only does it make it illegal to discriminate against persons with disabilities, public places and places of business are required by law to make accommodations for disabled persons. We must have handicapped access assistance tools in our public bathrooms. Wheelchair access must be made available. We cannot refuse service to an individual with a handicap or disability, even if providing such service or accommodation is costly.

Why, then, can we kill a human before he or she is born, on the basis of diminished ability, or disability, or handicap, especially if raising such a child will be costly—but we must accommodate all such individuals after they are born, no matter the cost? Make no mistake here: I think making those accommodations is the right thing to do. Killing those with potentially diminished abilities is wrong. The level of cognitive dissonance required to advocate for killing disabled people before they are born, but having to go to sometimes great lengths to care for them after they are born, is astounding.

While this has by no means been an exhaustive treatment of the ways in which we can address the arguments that support abortion rights, it does serve as a basic introduction to simple ways to refute some of the common varieties of abortion defenses. These include the "It's not a baby" argument, the "bodily autonomy" defense, "privacy" issues, the "poverty" issue, and the "No one wants a baby with diminished abilities" issue. There is, however, another fallacy which begs to be addressed.

Pro-life individuals will always encounter those who choose to deflect the issue by saying, "I am pro-life, but I am not going to tell anyone else what to do." Sadly, many in the clergy adopt this approach. While some who say this will be well-intentioned, others simply will not wish to discuss the issue and perhaps do not feel equipped to defend what they really believe. Perhaps they do not wish to offend and feel that such a position is neutral. There is a truth here at work though, and it is important. On real moral issues, there is no such thing as a neutral position. One can be neutral on whether or not to wear white after Labor Day, but an intellectually honest person cannot be neutral on whether or not it is appropriate to electively end the life of an unborn child simply because he or she is unwanted or inconvenient. In his essay[14] for the Christian Medical and Dental Society of Canada, Dr. John Patrick discusses the myth of moral neutrality. He says, "All societies share some fundamental ideas about what constitutes good and evil, *at least until they are in the terminal stages of social decay*" (emphasis added).

Dr. Patrick goes on to persuasively say the following: "The dominant modern approach stems from our own self-absorption. We say we create our own values. This is a seriously flawed theory because truth is made subservient to desire." He continues: "Creating our own values presumes that we can put ourselves in a kind of moral vacuum, but once there, we have no reason to create moral injunctions except those that satisfy our own desires." I submit to you that he is correct—any approach that tries to impose moral neutrality upon issues that clearly have moral implications is the beginning of chaos. In very eloquent terms, he goes on to tell us that, "The primary virtue of the morally neutral is tolerance. The question is, 'Can a society be built on the basis of tolerance?'" The answer to that is no. Are we expected to tolerate everything, no matter how unjust or harmful?

The "I am personally pro-life but I will not tell anyone else what to do" person fails to understand that this is not a justification of their neutrality. Almost 170 years ago, the Supreme Court was considering the question of slavery. Would the following statement find any agreement today? "I am personally against slavery, and have never owned slaves, but I am not going to tell anyone else what to do." In today's society, would a young man at a fraternity party who refuses to attempt to interfere in a sexual assault find any sympathy in the public eye by saying, "I am against rape, and have never raped anyone, but I wasn't about to tell anyone else what to do"? He would not find sympathy or agreement, and he should not. In any just and civil society, those who can speak and act in defense of those who cannot speak and act must do so—or they bear responsibility for what happens.

Dr. Patrick goes on to propose a starting list of four types of behaviors that should not be tolerated. His list of four, as a starting point, includes behaviors that are unloving, unjust, untruthful, and dishonorable. I submit to you that elective abortion on demand is all four. While Margaret Sanger said that the most merciful thing a large family can do to a young child is to kill it, I cannot fathom how anyone would agree with her on the basis that such behavior is loving. A modern abortion rights supporter has spoken publicly and claimed that her abortion was an act of love toward the child. This is simply not a rational point of view. There is nothing loving about ending the life of a helpless, innocent, and defenseless child because he or she is unwanted or inconvenient in some way. The only love expressed by an individual in this situation is love of self and love of lifestyle. There are very rare instances when a pregnancy must be ended before the child has a chance to survive after being delivered because the mother's life is truly in danger. This is also not something to be celebrated. From decades of personal experiences helping them, women in those rare situations don't celebrate anything and they certainly don't want to "shout" it. They mourn, deeply and often for years. They do not feel that what had to be done was loving—they feel that is was difficult and tragic. Elective abortion is also unjust. It is manifestly unjust to end the life of a child when there are other options. That child loses their life and all the choices and experiences that they would have enjoyed—and abortion does so without due process. In our constitutionally governed society, that is the very definition of unjust. Abortion on demand is also an untruthful institution. The very arguments presented and refuted earlier in this chapter, that the unborn is not a human person, that bodily autonomy justifies it, that privacy should allow it—those are all patently false statements.

Finally, abortion is a dishonorable industry. It is a cash cow for the owners of facilities and the physicians who perform them. The way in which women are persuaded that abortion is their best—indeed, their only—option is frankly outrageous. The fact that the world's largest corporate provider maintains its infrastructure with the assistance of tax dollars and then uses astounding amounts of money to buy the support of politicians, who in turn act to protect and advance the abortion agenda, is dishonorable. So are the political figures who accept blood money. You may have objections to the National Rifle Association and their lobbying choices, but the NRA does not receive tax dollars. Abortion is a huge financial enterprise—and when you take out the tax dollars Planned Parenthood receives, 80% of its remaining cash flow comes from abortion. Their repeated claims and assertions that "abortion is only 3% of what we do" are both untruthful and dishonorable.

While Dr. Patrick does not specifically address the "I am personally pro-life, but I will not tell anyone else what to do" person, his concluding paragraphs in this essay are appropriate for that individual to consider. He says, "Those who want a neutral policy usually say something like, 'You keep your opinions on morals private and I will do the same, and in that way we will both be happy.' This slick piece of sophistry is neither true nor honest.

The hidden implication is that there is no objective truth at stake—but as we have already seen, in order to have justice, objective truth is necessary." He is correct. I will now be somewhat less sophisticated than Dr. Patrick as I address this person directly: Educate yourself on the truth of abortion, then find your spine and pick a side.

I am certainly blessed in that I have as my wife a woman who is strong, wise, brilliant, thoughtful, and eloquent. I asked her to help me assemble the conclusion to this chapter, and she responded. She suggested that I point out that "Choosing to do nothing is choosing to do something." She is absolutely correct. When faced with what can legitimately be called evil, you can choose to oppose, or you can choose to support; but you can also choose to enable. Attempting a stance of neutrality on such an important issue is choosing to enable. Dietrich Bonhoeffer is well known for his stance against perhaps the greatest evil of the twentieth century—and for his stance he lost his life. He was frustrated by the unwillingness of the church to speak out against Nazi anti-Semitism. One of his most well-known quotes is this: "Silence in the face of evil is itself evil: God will not hold us guiltless. Not to speak is to speak. Not to act is to act." In a similar vein, British statesman Edmund Burke said, "All that is necessary for the triumph of evil is that good men do nothing."

Dear Reader—are you good? Are you willing to speak? Are you willing to act? Will you work to equip yourself to be good, to speak, and to act?

CHAPTER 5

MURDEROUS JURISPRUDENCE

"We are not final because we are infallible, but we are
infallible only because we are final."
Supreme Court Justice Robert Jackson, *Brown v. Allen,* 1953

The Constitution of the United States of America is a marvelous document. It is a testament to the brilliance of the Founders. It created the framework for the constitutional republic which we now have as the United States of America, a nation of, by, and for the people, grounded in democratic processes. We elect representatives whose responsibility is to serve in government. They then weigh issues in terms of what their constituents find to be important and what is important for the country as a whole.

We are not a pure "democracy." As such, we would be subject to mob rule—and that is one thing the Constitution was designed to prevent. We were not to be ruled by a king or a monarchy, but were intended to be governed by representatives who pass laws that are consistent with our Constitution and which respect the specific rights enumerated within that document. That is the function of the legislative branch of government. The executive branch has among its responsibilities the execution of that governance and the enforcement of our laws and the provision of our common defense. The judicial branch is responsible for the impartial handling of civil and criminal matters, as well as rendering decisions on the constitutionality of laws that are passed when citizens choose to dispute said laws as unjust or unconstitutional. The Supreme Court is the final authority on judicial matters, but it is not an infallible authority.

This chapter has significance in our cause to save vulnerable lives. For some readers, trying to understand legal terms makes your eyes glaze over. But try we must. Our goal is to respond with clarity regarding laws and ethics on the most pressing human rights issue of our time. To do so, the task ahead is to gain a baseline knowledge of how the U.S. legal system works— then survey an unfortunate history of poor judicial reasoning, half-truths, and outright lies that characterize rulings on abortion policy.

One legal term which you will hear when controversial matters are considered is the phrase *stare decisis*, which essentially translated from Latin means, "Let the decision stand." It is a concept in jurisprudence that is relied upon to protect prior judicial decisions, and to require that the court consider prior decisions on similar matters when rendering new decisions on aspects of the same topic. While *stare decisis* is an important part of judicial deliberations, it is not law and is not required to be followed in all matters. In fact, since the court heard *Van Staphorst v. Maryland* in 1791 as its first case, the Supreme Court of the United States has reversed itself more than 230 times.[15] *Stare decisis* is thus not a sacred inviolable principle; but supporters of *Roe v. Wade* would have you think that it is. For proof of that statement, all one must do is listen as pro-abortion senators interrogate judicial nominations made by Republican presidents and demand that they promise to adhere to *stare decisis*, especially as it regards *Roe v. Wade*.

The Supreme Court of the United States (SCOTUS) has made bad decisions before. Other than the decisions made on abortion, perhaps the most notoriously awful decision was *Dred Scott v. Sanford* in 1857. Dred Scott was an enslaved man who, along with his wife and daughters, was taken from a state in which slavery was legal into a state where it was not (in fact, into a territory which was not yet a state). He filed suit seeking his freedom, and that of his family. SCOTUS ruled against him and in favor of his owner. SCOTUS ruled in favor of slavery, at least in part, to try to settle the issue of slavery and achieve a political goal. They ruled in the 7-2 decision that no person of African ancestry could be a citizen and thus did not have standing to litigate anything, much less their own freedom. Instead of ruling on the rights of a human being, which are clearly enumerated within the Bill of Rights, they decided that this particular class of humanity (those of African descent) were deserving of no rights whatsoever. They ruled in favor of the slave owner, in part, because of the Fifth Amendment's protections against having property seized, because they determined that black people were property and not people.

No one alive today, with a rational mind and any sense of right and wrong, would defend *Dred Scott v. Sanford* today on the grounds of *stare decisis*, or any other grounds. Yet *Roe v. Wade*, also decided in a 7-2 decision, used some of the same arguments to justify abortion that were used to justify slavery. They made a decision which achieved the political goal of taking the regulation of abortion away from the states, with no regard whatsoever for the nature of the human life at stake in each and every abortion. In particular, they used the Fourteenth Amendment's supposed privacy protections and due process clauses to enable the abortion agenda and ignored the constitutional guarantees that no person could be deprived of life without due process of law. They did so by refusing to address the fact that the unborn person is a person. In fact, they feigned ignorance on this point.

Justice Harry Blackmun, author of the majority opinion in *Roe*, wrote as if the nature of the unborn was not known at the time. He specifically said that "If this suggestion of personhood is established, the appellant's case, of course, collapses, for the fetus' right to life would then be guaranteed specifically by the Amendment."[16] He was referencing the Fourteenth Amendment, and stated that his conclusion was "that the word 'person,' as used in the Fourteenth Amendment, does not include the unborn." He provided no reason that justified or legitimized that ruling.

At the time *Roe* was decided, medicine lacked the ultrasound technology we have today. Rapidly available and sensitive hormone tests like the human chorionic gonadotropin (HCG) also were not available. We can now easily obtain a real-time dynamic assessment of the viability, of the living condition, of each and every unborn child. That was not possible in 1973. Justice Blackmun was able to construct the majority opinion because of that ignorance, making *Roe* a decision founded upon and protected by ignorance. We can no longer plead ignorance, so abortion's supporters must rely on *stare decisis,* and they fight against any reconsideration of *Roe's* injustice based on the undeniable evidence we have that the unborn cannot be legitimately and rationally considered to be anything other than a human person.

In a society of more than 300 million people, there will inevitably be situations where the rights of one individual or group will come into conflict with the rights of other individuals or groups. It is the responsibility of SCOTUS to rule properly and fairly on such conflicts, and to decide which individual or group has the most to lose in any such conflict. It is safe to say that life itself is the most important human right. Life is the first right listed as a protected liberty in the Declaration of Independence, and it can and should be argued that all other rights must be subservient to that right.

We have a right to religious expression, but that right is not allowed to endanger or take the life of another. Laws against the unregulated handling of venomous snakes have stood against legal challenges because life can be endangered, despite cults that consider snake handling a religious rite. Religions that call for the execution of individuals caught in certain sins are not allowed to exercise that belief, unless their adherents otherwise break the law and face the consequences.

We have freedom of speech—but we cannot yell "Fire" in a crowded theater, without risking a penalty for endangering people in the melee that might ensue. The exercise of constitutionally protected liberties is not allowed when the exercise of those liberties endangers the lives or takes the lives of others, as the right to life itself is paramount. Any "liberty" that takes an innocent life without due process is no liberty at all but is, instead, a tyranny. We also have freedom of the press but we are not allowed to print things that we know are not true in order to harm another individual—if we do, we can be charged with slander and libel.

In order, then, for rights to due process and privacy to be used to justify abortion rights, the unborn baby's identity as a human person must be denied. There is no medical or scientific basis for justifying such a practice. Any argument that chooses a point during pregnancy when life begins—at any point other than conception—is an arbitrary argument lacking reason, science, and logic. It is intended solely for the achievement of a political and/or social goal. Any statement that "we cannot know when life begins" is a ludicrous and dishonest statement. We know when life begins and we know when it ends. There are quantifiable scientific measures that establish these points as fact. The question, then, is not when does life begin, but when should a living person be considered worthy of constitutional protections. Science, objective reason, and logic fail to give us a reason to choose any point other than conception for the designation of life and personhood and constitutional protections. Any choice of any point otherwise is a choice to discriminate against one individual and take their life in order to obtain some perceived benefit for another individual. When the rights of different individuals come into conflict, with one individual's life being on the line, justice demands ruling with the individual whose life is at risk.

It is vital to understand what the SCOTUS has said about abortion in order to understand the state in which we find ourselves. An excellent summation of the essential facts can be found on the webpage of a group called Abort73 (www.abort73.com). In my research, I also discovered an organization called the Personhood Alliance (www.personhood.org).

In 1973, SCOTUS ruled on two cases, one from Texas and one from Georgia. The Texas case was *Roe v. Wade* and involved the case of a woman named Norma McCorvey, who was given the pseudonym Jane Roe in her case against the Dallas County District Attorney Henry Wade. She was a single woman with an unplanned pregnancy who lacked the resources to travel to a state in which she could obtain an abortion legally. According to her lawyers, she sought to prevent Wade from enforcing a law preventing her ability to obtain an abortion in Texas. The length of time it took for the case to make its way through the judicial process was longer than the pregnancy, and she delivered her child and placed her for adoption. She later regretted the fact that her name and her situation were used by abortion advocates to advance the cause of abortion. McCorvey became a prolific pro-life activist, openly and repeatedly calling for the overturn of *Roe*. She died in 2017.

The Georgia case of *Doe v. Bolton* involved a woman named Sandra Cano, a young mother of three. Her pseudonym of Mary Doe was used by attorney Margie Pitts Hames to pursue a challenge against Arthur Bolton, the attorney general of Georgia at the time. Georgia law allowed abortion only under very limited circumstances, and then, only for residents of Georgia. Cano later claimed that Hames lied to her so that she would have a plaintiff. The young mother did not really seek or desire an abortion, and the material facts of her case were misrepresented by Hames. Like McCorvey, Cano fought until her death in 2014 to see the ruling that bears her name overturned. *Roe* and *Doe* were the first two major rulings on abortion by the Supreme Court and were both handed down on the same day: January 22, 1973.

In *Roe,* the Court ruled based on their interpretation of the Fourteenth Amendment that the states only had a "compelling" interest in protecting the life of the unborn after a threshold of "viability." They arbitrarily set this marker at twenty-eight weeks, which is the beginning of the third trimester. This invalidated any law in any of the fifty states that prohibited or regulated abortion prior to twenty-eight weeks. They went further and ruled that abortion would be permissible in the third trimester if the woman's life was in danger.

In *Doe,* they struck down most of Georgia's laws regulating access to abortion and struck down the residency requirement. They ruled that danger to the maternal life was not the only thing that would justify abortion, but that a broad definition of "health" was to be used. This essentially allows an abortionist and the patient to say anything they wish to justify the termination of the pregnancy. Majority opinion author Justice Harry Blackmun wrote that the health exemption would take into consideration "physical, emotional, psychological, (and) familial" conditions and that doing so would allow "the attending physician the room he needs to make his best medical judgment." Stated alternatively, and more accurately, if the woman claims that the pregnancy is physically uncomfortable, or emotionally distressing, or psychologically depressing, or financially or relationally difficult—then the inconvenient child can be killed with no consideration of his or her humanity.

The next time SCOTUS visited the issue was 1976 in *Planned Parenthood of Missouri v. Danforth*. John Danforth was the Attorney General of the state of Missouri. In this decision, SCOTUS struck down Missouri laws which required parental consent for abortions for minors and required spousal consent for abortion for married couples. The Court ruled that since the state had no standing to prohibit abortion, especially in the first trimester, that the parents of a minor also could not be allowed to prohibit abortion. Similarly, they ruled that since the state could not prohibit abortion, a husband and father of the child whose life was at stake also had no standing to veto the abortion.

While there are still some states which require parental consent, each of these states have some means of what is known as "judicial bypass" to allow a minor to obtain an abortion without her parents' consent or even their knowledge. These "judicial bypasses" were codified in 1990 in the cases of *Hodgson v. Minnesota* and *Ohio v. Akron Center for Reproductive Health*. Abortion facilities always have an attorney and a judge on standby to obtain the necessary bypass for minors who seek abortion services and do not wish to notify parents. It is a mind-numbingly stupid dichotomy to say that a school nurse cannot dispense a tablet of Tylenol to a student without written permission from a parent—but that the same nurse can take a minor to an abortion clinic during school hours, in order to conceal the abortion from parents. The strength of the bodily autonomy argument is insufficient to overcome our restrictions on minors getting tattoos or buying tobacco, but we are intended to allow it to justify abortion without parental knowledge or consent.

It was another ten years before the next case came before SCOTUS. In 1986, SCOTUS heard *Thornburgh v. American College of Obstetricians and*

Gynecologists. Dick Thornburgh was the governor of Pennsylvania and this case involved the opposition by the American College of Obstetricians and Gynecologists (ACOG) to Pennsylvania's Abortion Control Act of 1982. This legislation clearly stated the interest that the legislature in Pennsylvania had in protecting life, in requiring informed consent and a waiting period, and other meaningful regulations in regard to abortion. President Ronald Reagan had sought a case to bring about a challenge to *Roe,* and there was hope that this case would have been it. In the majority opinion, written again by Justice Harry Blackmun, the state's numerous restrictions on abortion were struck down. These restrictions were what most reasonable people would conclude were common-sense restrictions on abortion. There was a provision for a standard informed consent process which would inform the woman of the risks of the procedure, the alternatives to the procedure, the availability of resources to assist her if she chose to parent, and aspects of fetal development appropriate to the gestational age of the pregnancy.

Remember from our earlier discussion of informed consent that professional and ethical medical standards require informed consent, before procedures, that cover risks and alternatives and the implications of any proposed procedures. This is a professional standard to which all physicians who perform surgical procedures are held. However, in the case of abortion, the court decided that such restrictions were illegitimate as they were an effort by the state to "intimidate women into continuing their pregnancies." Abortion supporters have always been desperate to have abortion considered to be legitimate health care. Yet this case is one of the earliest and most prominent examples of how they always seek to have abortion exempted from the professional standards to which all of legitimate medicine is held. The Pennsylvania law also would have codified a medical record keeping requirement similar to that which is expected of legitimate medicine, and would have required that abortionists be prepared to render care and aid to infants who were not yet dead upon delivery. The abortionist push for infanticide protections actually began with this case in 1986.

Then, in the 1989 case of *Webster v. Reproductive Health Services*, SCOTUS, for the first time, began to re-evaluate *Roe*. In this case, the 5-4 majority let a Missouri statute stand. That statute declared that life begins at conception and acknowledged problems with *Roe*. They stated that "*Roe's* rigid trimester analysis has proved to be unsound in principle and unworkable in practice. In such circumstances, this Court does not refrain from reconsidering prior constitutional rulings, notwithstanding *stare decisis*." It went on to say that the "framework's key elements—trimesters and viability—are not found in the Constitution's text," and then that "There is also no reason why the State's compelling interest in protecting potential human life should not extend throughout pregnancy rather than coming into existence only at the point of viability." Justice Sandra Day O'Connor left the door open to carefully re-examine *Roe* when the constitutionality of a state statute is in question because of *Roe*. Justice Antonin Scalia made his conviction that *Roe* was bad jurisprudence clear when he stated that that *Roe's* validity was questionable because it was "broader-than-required-by-the-facts." Sadly, while this all sounds like a victory for life, it had little effect in practice.

The next case, in 1992, was *Planned Parenthood v. Casey*. In this case, the court largely did away with the trimester framework of *Roe*. Instead, SCOTUS adopted a "viability" concept that ignored one of the two ways in which the term "viability" is used in obstetric medical practice. *Casey* came to the court because Planned Parenthood once again challenged Pennsylvania law regarding abortion. This decision was a mixed bag. The Court actually ignored *stare decisis* as it relates to prior abortion precedents and overruled its own 1976 decision to invalidate parental consent requirements, record-keeping requirements, and informed consent; it also allowed a brief mandatory waiting period. Sadly, however, the opinion that *Roe* had no constitutional basis whatsoever held by Justices William Rehnquist, Byron White, Antonin Scalia, and Clarence Thomas did not win the day.

Abortion not only maintained its inappropriate constitutional protection; now, the trimester framework was disallowed, and states were prevented from restricting abortion prior to the gestational age at which an unborn child might survive if delivered. States would still be required to permit abortion after that point if the mother's "health" was deemed to be at risk. This is now the standard against which any pro-life legislation must be crafted, and it focuses on the concept of "viability." As discussed in an earlier chapter, this assessment of viability is not one which should be used to determine life or personhood. In the most accurate medical terms, it is simply a *prognostic* assessment for the potential for continued life if delivered and is not in any way a *diagnostic* assessment of whether or not the child is alive or is a person.

The final two cases I will discuss in this chapter involve notorious late-term abortionist Leroy Carhart. He is a physician best known for his willingness to perform late-term abortions on nearly full-term babies. He has been considered a heroic champion of the abortion movement, having been given awards by NARAL and Planned Parenthood. He chose to challenge restrictions on a particular method of abortion known as intact dilation and extraction, also known as partial-birth abortion. This is an abortion method in which a pregnancy is well past the gestational age at which the child can survive. It requires that labor be induced. When the patient is nearly fully dilated and almost ready to push, the child is manipulated into a breech or feet-first position and then the legs and buttocks and body are pulled out. Then, before the head delivers and the child is born alive, a sharp instrument, usually scissors, is pushed up into the head through the base of the skull at the back of the child's neck. A suction instrument is then inserted into the hole, which has been brutally created while the baby is still alive and can feel everything, and the brain is suctioned out, allowing the skull to collapse and ensuring that the baby is born dead. This procedure is never necessary from a medical point of view. As it still requires labor, it does not accelerate the delivery of a child when time is critical because the mother is ill. Induction of labor without killing the baby is just as fast in terms of achieving a delivery, and a Cesarean section is much faster.

You must understand the background regarding efforts to outlaw this particularly brutal and medically unnecessary procedure. In 1996, Congress passed a ban on partial-birth abortion. President Clinton wanted to veto the measure but did not have medical cover to do so. At the time, the American College of Obstetricians and Gynecologists had a position statement that accurately stated that such a procedure was not necessary to protect the woman's life or health. Clinton could not veto the bill based on its lack of a health exception when the largest medical organization of OB/GYNs held the position that it was not necessary to protect the woman's health. Enter Clinton's Associate White House Counsel, future SCOTUS Justice Elena Kagan. The wording of the ACOG position on the issue at the time said that ACOG "could identify no circumstances under which this procedure…would be the only option to save the life or preserve the health of the woman." A review of documents from her time in the Clinton White House shows that Kagan gave ACOG the wording which, when used by ACOG, would change their public position on the issue and would give Clinton the medical cover needed to veto the bill. She ignored sound medical conclusions and data and persuaded ACOG to change its public position on the issue in a way which would allow the President to veto the ban.[17] As a result of ACOG's withdrawal of an accurate piece of medical literature, Clinton issued his veto and pretended to be very upset about having to protect such a horrific procedure.

The state of Nebraska then passed a ban on partial-birth abortion, and Dr. Leroy Carhart challenged it in court. The court heard the case and issued its opinion in a 5-4 vote that struck down the Nebraska ban which had been defended by Nebraska attorney general Don Stenberg. The four dissenting Justices were Rehnquist, Scalia, Thomas, and Kennedy. (Notice that, over the years, the makeup of the court has changed; what was almost always a 7-2 vote to protect abortion became a 5-4 vote with vigorous and well-reasoned dissent.)

Then in 2003, the 108th Congress once again enacted a ban on partial-birth abortion and President George W. Bush signed it without hesitation. Predictably, it was challenged in court and once again Dr. Carhart was the challenger. This time, in *Gonzales v. Carhart,* a 5-4 decision of the court ignored *stare decisis* and reversed itself on *Stenberg v. Carhart.* The majority opinion found that the new ban enacted by the 108th Congress corrected the vagaries of language that were part of the problem with Nebraska's ban that was stricken down in *Stenberg.* In a concurring opinion, Justices Thomas and Scalia reiterated their conviction that *Roe* and *Casey* were not proper interpretations of the Constitution and should be reconsidered.

What can we glean from a study of these cases? First, the makeup of the court has changed. Second, there are examples of the court reversing itself on the issue of abortion, especially as science and knowledge have advanced and as highly specific arguments are presented to the court. This should serve as an admonition to state legislative bodies who wish to change what is currently interpreted as constitutional—an admonition that they should heed by taking the obligation to protect all persons very seriously and soberly. Casual legislation will not work. Thoughtful study and deliberation should occur, as pro-life advocates muster the courage required to accomplish the lofty and laudable goal of reversing the worst SCOTUS precedent in history.

What should be the basis of further legislative efforts? SCOTUS has, at times, had as many as four Justices who together have held that *Roe* has no constitutional basis whatsoever. The court has also reversed itself before on the issue of abortion, as outlined above. Specifically, in *Gonzales v. Carhart*, the court reversed itself and upheld a ban on partial-birth abortion when it had previously stricken down a ban on the same procedure in *Stenberg v. Carhart*. What made the difference? The federal ban on partial-birth abortion addressed the issue with a higher degree of medical specificity. It is my strongly held conviction that any successful effort to overturn *Roe* must address the issue of life with medical and scientific accuracy and specificity, and must also bring the issue of personhood into the equation. This would force the judicial system to re-evaluate the injustice of using the constitutional protections of due process and privacy for one individual's preferences to disenfranchise another individual of their right to life itself.

CHAPTER 6

FAILURE: HOW THE CHURCH CONTINUES TO ACHIEVE IT

Dr. Bernard Nathanson, essentially the father of the abortion movement in the early 1970s, once revealed the secret of his success. The reason that supporters of abortion rights were able to accomplish so much with *Roe v. Wade*, he said, was that the church was asleep. In many ways, the church has remained asleep on this issue. "Leaders" in the church say that they cannot talk about political issues—on that, they are gravely mistaken. The IRS regulations that grant churches tax-exempt status only forbid the endorsement of a specific political candidate by a church. There are no regulations regarding the discussion of issues like abortion. There is currently nothing in the law or in IRS regulations which would allow a church to be penalized for speaking on the issue of abortion.

Far too many church leaders are afraid to speak about controversial subjects. They fear negative publicity and offending members of their congregation who are on the opposite side of the issue. Perhaps I am mistaken, but isn't it a pastor's responsibility to speak truth, guard his flock, and keep them from harm? Abortion, the shedding of innocent blood, the intentional taking of human life, is an abomination in God's eyes. It is not the responsibility of the priest or the pastor to designate abortion as sin—God already did. While the church has been asleep and unwilling to address the issue with anything remotely resembling vigor, more than sixty million babies have perished. Far too many in the church have no awareness of the issue at all. The Word tells us that "My people are destroyed from lack of knowledge"—especially true in the case of abortion, where the innocent blood of babies who have perished is on our hands. In fact, Hosea 4:6 has what could be interpreted as a dire warning for pastors and preachers who don't want to touch the issue of abortion. Consider the text: "My people are destroyed from lack of knowledge. Because you have rejected knowledge, I also reject you as my priests; because you have ignored the law of your God, I also will ignore your children." To whom is God speaking? The priests, the leaders of His people. Who are the modern-day priests? Pastors and priests, that's who.

Jesus also addressed the issue of speaking out and directed his criticism to the Pharisaical religious leaders of the day. As Jesus and his disciples were entering the city of Jerusalem, the disciples were praising God and worshipping Him. The Pharisees wanted them to be silent, and in Luke 19:39-41, Jesus responds: "But some of the Pharisees in the crowd said to Him, 'Teacher, rebuke your disciples!' 'I tell you,' He answered, 'if they remain silent the very stones will cry out.' As Jesus approached Jerusalem and saw the city, He wept over it." You might ask, "How does that apply to abortion?" It should be obvious. We have far too many leaders in the American church today who do not wish to address issues such as abortion. They fear criticism. They fear loss of members who might not agree with a Biblical message. And they lack the courage and the wisdom to address a difficult issue. Or perhaps they are on the wrong side of the issue altogether. Regardless, oftentimes when a congregant approaches a pastor and asks about seeing abortion addressed from the pulpit, they are told that such social and controversial issues will not be addressed—that it is not the role of the church to speak to those issues. This is similar to the Pharisaical rebuke of the noise being made by the disciples.

We are at a tipping point in America today on the issue of abortion. On one side, radical leftists are pushing an agenda that seeks to end all restrictions on abortion. They even allow the murder of children born alive when the abortion procedure was unsuccessful, and are also pushing for all conscience protections to be removed. These protections are in place to protect health care providers from being forced to perform or participate in abortions, as well as to protect religious institutions from having to pay for abortion through the health coverage they may provide to individuals. On the other side, many state legislatures have become more active in their fight to protect the unborn and are crafting legislation that they hope will challenge what is currently considered to be constitutional on the issue of abortion. We are seeing a surge in grassroots involvement in this issue. Where the church should have led and didn't, individuals and non-church groups are doing so—fulfilling what Jesus said about seeing "the very stones cry out."

The sins of the church on this issue are many. The leaders of the church are, among other things, called to be watchmen. When society was wrestling with the abortion issue prior to *Roe* in 1973, the watchmen were asleep. They didn't sound the clarion call about the impending danger. They didn't want to get involved or didn't even realize that they needed to be. Too many remain asleep, or afraid, or uninterested. Too many choose to ignore the mandate to be salt and light. Oh, there are some churches who contribute small sums to local crisis pregnancy centers. A few churches have counseling ministries that serve post-abortive women and men. A small number are actively involved in the issue in other ways. But there are not very many churches in which you will often hear abortion discussed in more than a passing way from the pulpit, and then only once in a blue moon. There are not very many who will even give the time of day to pro-life activists or to the directors of pro-life pregnancy centers. I am the medical director of the pregnancy center in our town and am close friends with the executive director who founded the center thirty-five years ago. I know, from my own experience and from hers, the frustrating level of difficulty encountered when we try to move local churches on this issue. And there were far too few churches who gave the recent movie *Unplanned* even a mention—what a missed opportunity!

The failures of the church to be more active on this issue, to encourage members' involvement in the electoral process, and to educate members are not the only ways in which the church has failed and continues to fail on this issue. The way that the church has treated women who are unmarried and pregnant, and the way they have treated post-abortive women is also tragic.

One in four women sitting in church on any given Sunday morning is post-abortive—and the vast majority have few individuals, if any, in their lives who know about it. Why have so many unwed women in the church felt that abortion was their best option? Because, as women in the church with an unplanned pregnancy consider abortion, the two most common expectations they have if they were to discuss their pregnancy with a church leader is that he would be judgmental or condemning. More than half of women surveyed agree that their church does not have a ministry prepared to discuss options during an unplanned pregnancy. When the church fails to address an issue, you better believe the world will discuss it. Other solid statistics tell us that 70% of women who have had an abortion in America list their religious preference as Christian. Additionally, 35% of women who have had an abortion indicate that they attend church weekly, and 36% say that at the time of their abortion they were attending church at least once a month or more. The church's failure on this is multi-faceted.

First, most men and women who grew up in church did not receive Bible-based teaching and instruction on sex, love, relationships, and marriage. They were never taught about the beauty, purpose, and importance of sex within the boundaries God proscribes. As I shared earlier, my zeal on this issue is born from my own difficult mistakes in this regard. Churches must speak to both genders, as it takes two to make a baby. They almost certainly heard about the "rules," but they never had their "why" questions answered. They were never told that sexual abstinence until marriage gives a couple the best chance at the lowest divorce rate. They were never told in a convincing way that treating sex casually makes it less meaningful, damaging their ability to bond deeply and intimately. They were never told that God's instructions about sex were not meant to deprive us of something fun but were intended to show us the best way. God's instructions about sexual activity were treated like a prison fence and punishment instead of being clearly demonstrated to be more like guard rails on a mountain road—there for our safety and to help us reach our destination.

Second, the way the church and its membership at large has commonly treated the Christian woman with an unplanned pregnancy is problematic. One would think that being pregnant and unmarried is the absolute worst thing a woman could do. They are made to feel shame at every turn. They know that as the pregnancy progresses, there will be all those sidelong glances and hushed whispers every time she walks by. "Did you see her?" "What nerve for her to come here!" "Her parents must be so ashamed." And then there are those who criticize her parents as well, which only compounds her shame and guilt. Did you know that if churched women stopped having abortions, the abortion industry would lose $250,000,000 annually?

Nothing is more effective in driving the churchgoing, unwed, pregnant woman into the abortion clinic waiting room than the reactions that those in the church have historically had to unwed, pregnant women. The church has been unwilling to follow the example Jesus set when the woman caught in sexual sin was brought before him by a group of Pharisaical, judgmental men that wanted to stone her to death. Jesus showed wisdom when he called them to account for their own sin—and compassion when he reached down, took her hand to help her up, and counseled her to "sin no more" (John 8:11). The Bible teaches that sexual activity outside of marriage is a sin, but it never says that being pregnant is a sin. The church has elevated sexual sin to a level that is worse than gluttony, jealousy, greed, envy, lying, gossip, and stealing—but that is not a Biblical doctrine. The unwed, pregnant woman has been driven to the abortion clinic because she thought she had no choice. She has been left to suffer in shame and silence with her guilt and regret; and so have the post-abortive fathers of these children.

This brings us to a third vital point. Leaders in the church have rarely made post-abortive counseling a priority, if they even offer it at all. Most churches will have some excellent general counseling ministries, but few have any focus at all on the needs of post-abortive parishioners. God never intended the church to be a place for perfect people—He intended it to be a place for people to be in community, grow together, and care for one another's needs. He intended it to be a place where the hurting find healing. Imagine a church world in which the pastor focuses on abortion with this attitude: "If you're unmarried and find yourself pregnant, don't go to the abortion clinic. Come to the church! We will help you with the pregnancy. We will help you learn to be a good parent, or we will help you through the adoption process. Come to the church! We love you and we love your baby! Have you had an abortion and now are struggling? Come to the church!

There is love, grace, mercy, redemption, and healing here! Come to the church! We will help you be healed, and then enable you to help heal others! Come to the church!" That is the Kingdom perspective on this issue—but sadly, the church world and the Kingdom are rarely the same thing. They are supposed to be the same, but in America, far too often, they are not.

How does this begin to change? We Christians must insist that this issue be made a priority. Do not take no for an answer. If you have a pastor who is reluctant to tackle what is perhaps the biggest ministry issue in the church today, get a new pastor or find a new church. Pastors, if you really are serious about doing the right thing, start by educating yourself. "My people are destroyed from lack of knowledge." God said it, I'm just quoting Him. "How can I do that?" You should be asking that question if you are a pastor. There is an easy answer. Care Net (www.care-net.org) is a professional organization of Christian-led pregnancy centers currently with 1,714 affiliated centers. Every state in the Union has multiple centers. Care Net centers are devoted to providing services that empower women with unplanned or crisis pregnancies to make good choices for themselves and their families. They serve their communities with excellence and love. Isn't that supposed to be what the church is doing? With the geographic distribution of these centers across the country, it would be hard to find a pastor who would have to drive more than an hour to find a Care Net affiliate. The directors of these centers often have little, if any, support or assistance from many churches, and most directors would be thrilled to have the pastoral staff of any church come, learn, and discover what they can do to advance the Kingdom of God on the issue of abortion. Heartbeat International (www.heartbeatinternational.org) is another umbrella organization with over 2,600 centers around the world, and then there are many centers that are not affiliated with either organization. No one can say that they cannot find a center near them.

Discuss the issue of meeting the needs of post-abortive members with your ministry staff. There are a number of excellent training programs which can be completed by ministry teams quickly, of which one of the best is *Surrendering The Secret*. The curriculum of a program like this brings healing and restoration to the most broken places, in which many people find themselves. Far too many have given up hope in ever being healed and whole again. *Surrendering The Secret* is time tested and proven, used by many pregnancy centers that provide post-abortive ministry.

Here is a challenge to all pastors who read these words. It's instructive how the Passion Translation paraphrases Romans 1:20: "From the creation of the world… [God] has made his wonderful attributes easily perceived, for seeing the visible makes us understand the invisible. So then, this leaves everyone without excuse." Now that you know where you can go to see what you need to see and learn what you need to learn, you have no excuse.

I am not demanding that pastors financially support pregnancy centers. Many pastors are unwilling to meet with pregnancy center directors because that is what they think that the directors are seeking. While financial support will always be welcome—indeed, needed since virtually all these centers are nonprofit organizations that function on the generosity of their communities—there is so much more to this issue than the money. One of your primary obligations as a pastor is to teach, train, and equip your flock to function in this world that is only our temporary home. To do that, you must understand this issue and then act accordingly.

Pastors must become more willing to be involved on this issue. Standing firmly against the institutionalized murder of innocent children must be considered a Kingdom issue. In spring 2019, in the Tennessee General Assembly, there was a valiant effort to pass legislation that used unarguable medical proof of when life begins that linked viability with the beginning of a baby's heartbeat. It combined that evidence with novel constitutional arguments that have never been presented to a federal court, in an effort to come against *Roe v. Wade*. It failed for a variety of reasons, many of which will be discussed in the next chapter. My reasons for being so disappointed in the church were poignantly highlighted at a press conference that preceded a Senate floor vote that did not go well for the bill. During the work on this bill, many faithful, sincere Christians devoted much time and energy to speaking to legislators and to organizing grassroots support. However, the number of pastors whose involvement I witnessed can be counted on the fingers of one hand, without using all of the fingers.

We held a press conference to show the broad support this proposed legislation enjoyed across the state, and only four pastors were there. No additional pastors joined later to sit in the Senate gallery during the vote. I am aware of no other pastors who contacted members of the Senate to discuss this issue. We were painfully aware, however, of the more than forty supporters of Planned Parenthood who stood outside the Senate chamber chanting, "Thank God for legal abortion." There were more than ten times as many people there invoking the name of God to support the atrocity of abortion as there were pastors there to support a true, Biblical position on the issue. My wife and I left the Capitol that day with a terrible fear for where the church is at today. Eight of thirty-three senators voted in a way that supported the proposed legislation that day. Of the twenty-five who did not, I wonder how many were contacted by their own pastors beforehand and urged to show their support. I wonder how many were reminded of the importance of having their actions line up with their words. Three senators even used Scripture and cited Biblical references as they reminded us all of their pro-life credentials... then told us all their reasons for voting against advancing this important legislation. How many of them have pastors who will have called them to account?

One of my closest friends is a pastor. He is one of the ones who was at the press conference, and he is definitely an exception in the world of today's pastors. He is bold and fierce on this and other issues. His name is Lyndon B. Allen, and you should see what his perspective is by getting his book, *Total Life Victory*. Lyndon is fond of quoting nineteenth century pastor and evangelist Charles Finney. Finney was part of the revival known as the Second Great Awakening, which is generally considered to have run from the 1820s to the 1850s. This period of revival is credited for a number of things, which include the birth of the anti-slavery movement and the women's rights movement, as well as the beginning of the Salvation Army and the YMCA. Finney said, in regard to the involvement of Christians in the political process, "The time has come that Christians must vote for honest men and take consistent ground in politics or the Lord will curse them...Christians have been exceedingly guilty in this matter. But the time has come when they must act differently...Christians seem to act as if they thought God did not see what they do in politics. But I tell you He does see it—and He will bless or curse this nation according to the course they Christians take in politics." He also said, "If Satan rules in our halls of legislation—the pulpit is responsible for it. If our politics become so corrupt that the very foundations of our government are ready to fall away—the pulpit is responsible for it."

Another pastor whose messages I respect, Pastor Allen Jackson of World Outreach Church in Murfreesboro, Tennessee, echoes these themes. He has said, "The only thing to which evil will yield is a force greater than itself." Why has abortion, the institutionalized killing of unwanted innocent helpless human beings, enjoyed such success in the decades since *Roe*? Because it has not yet encountered a force greater than itself. God put the church on earth to be that force, and sadly the church has yet to find its way on this issue. It is time for that to change, and for pastors like Lyndon Allen and Allen Jackson to take the lead. Our culture is desperately in need of salt and light on this issue, and the church must be willing to step up to the Biblical mandate to be salt and light.

When one examines Scripture, one will not be able to find a silent prophet or leader. No one was ever nicknamed "The Silent Prophet" or "The Quiet King." What you will find is a lengthy and distinguished list of prophets and leaders who were not afraid to speak truth to people, including those in power. Moses was initially reluctant to speak, but became one of Israel's most important leaders because he did speak in spite of his reluctance. Samuel, Nathan, Ezra, Nehemiah, Isaiah, Jeremiah, Ezekiel, Daniel, Hosea, Joel, Amos, and others all were bold in addressing the issues of the day. Each of the Apostles were bold, even in the face of death. Will any pastor today face death because he speaks about life? Almost certainly not… yet far too many act as if they would. Jeremiah, in particular, is known for having an unpopular message. He even wrote an entire book named for the sadness of the state of things—it is called Lamentations. In the book which bears his name, he talks of how God's Word and God's name are burned upon his heart, and how he was compelled to speak about issues. In Jeremiah 20:9, he says, "But if I say 'I will not mention His word or speak anymore in His name,' His Word is in my heart like a fire, a fire shut up in my bones. I am weary of holding it in; indeed, I cannot."

How many of our pastors in the church in America today have Him or His Word so deeply burned into their hearts that they feel compelled to speak about issues, especially the issue of the ongoing slaughter of thousands of unborn bearers of the *Imago Dei* each and every day? How many are sufficiently weary of holding it in that they are ready to become standard-bearers on this issue? If they are unwilling to speak about life, do they really have that fire in their hearts and in their bones that comes from truly possessing God's Word within them? When the church is silent, evil advances and society deteriorates.

Consider the church in Germany during the years leading up to World War II and during the Holocaust. Most were silent in the face of pure and unadulterated evil. In a few short years, the Nazis exterminated six million Jews and five million others—Gypsies, homosexuals, political dissidents, and the very few Christian leaders like Dietrich Bonhoeffer who were willing to speak. In his book about the Holocaust, *How Do You Kill 11 Million People*, author Andy Andrews makes the point that in order to do something so atrocious, you must lie about it—at least, at first.

The Nazis lied—about their intentions, and about the humanity of those they sought to exterminate. They referred to Jews as *untermensch*, a word which means "less than human." That sounds eerily similar to the talking points used by supporters of abortion when they refer to babies in the womb. A Democratic pundit recently stated, with a substantial amount of vigor, that when a woman is pregnant, it is not a human being she is carrying. The unborn are called blobs of tissue, clots of blood, clumps of cells— anything but a baby—because the lie is necessary to dull the senses, deceive the ignorant, and achieve their purpose. Who in society should be the first to be a standard-bearer of truth? We cannot expect our political leaders to do that. Who then should it be? The church. Was the church a standard bearer of truth opposing Nazi propaganda in the 1930s and 1940s? No, they were not. Has the church in America been a standard bearer of truth on abortion? Largely, no. Sadly, no. Tragically, no.

Consider the story of a small church positioned along the railroad tracks that led to Auschwitz, the notorious death camp in which millions were gassed to death and then cremated. (Incidentally, the Nazis treated the corpses of their victims with more dignity than the abortion industry does. They cremated the vast majority of the remains of their victims. The abortion industry just fought against an Indiana law that requires that infant remains from abortions be buried or cremated—and they took that battle all the way to the Supreme Court, instead of simply accepting a requirement that they handle fetal remains properly.) With predictable German promptness and timing, a trainload full of Jews bound destined for the slaughter passed this little church every Sunday morning during the hours of worship.

The tracks were so close to the church that the congregants inside could hear the fearful cries and wailing of the Jews who were about to die. What was the church's response? They chose to "sing a little louder," according to some who were there and told the story of their shame later. They chose to ignore the plight of innocents destined for a brutal and unjust death. Rather than act on the distressing knowledge of what was happening, they sang louder in order to avoid having to think about what they were hearing. Is the church in America now doing the same thing? We have far more ability to do something in the here and now about abortion than the church in Germany was able to do there and then. The question is, are we?

Abortion is not the only issue in which the church in America has been reluctant to enter the fray. Racial injustice is another such issue. While many churches have begun to confess and confront racism in intentional ways, we could be doing better. Responding to racial injustice rightfully deserves its own book. An article in *The Christian Chronicle*[18] discussed a book titled *Eerie Silence* written by Amman Saheli—a black minister for the West Oakland Church of Christ. He grew up in San Francisco. A highly educated man, he says that his book is a plea for people of faith to speak out against injustice and to "truly embrace the radical love of Jesus that protects and cherishes all of humanity." He outlines not only the horrors of slavery but also the injustice of Jim Crow laws—and many aspects of racial discrimination that continue to effect U.S. society today. He refers to feeling like Jeremiah did as a reaction to the silence on important issues. Saheli criticizes the church by saying, "We talk about being like the first-century Christians, but we espouse an American version of that vision that says 'be silent' on divisive issues, on issues of race."

He could not be more accurate, and his statement is also true of abortion. Christians are called to stand up for the equality and value of every life. Both racism and abortion are sins the church has long ignored. When bringing up either one of these glaring blind spots that afflict American Christianity, be prepared to encounter every excuse, partisan knee-jerk reaction, and resolute attempts by fellow believers to change the subject. Saheli also says, "No one alive today created the concept and context of race and racism, but we are currently responsible for interrupting, disrupting, and dismantling its soul-crushing effects." His words are also applicable to the responsibility that the church has in regard to abortion. He accurately describes the state of the church on such issues as a state of "cognitive dissonance," seeing injustice but acting like you do not. He reminds us that Jesus demonstrated concern for the marginalized, oppressed, and the least of these. In this, he is also correct. Bravo, Amman Saheli, bravo.

I am weary of pastors and ministry leaders who speak of a desire to see revival in America but who will not involve themselves on the issues that cause us to desire revival, indeed to desperately need revival. In looking at six different periods thought to have been revivals in the last three hundred years, one commonality that emerges is good leadership by those unafraid of speaking to the issues of the day. Each of those revivals enlarged the church, won souls to the kingdom, and often improved society and culture as a whole.

From prayer, studying the Bible, and dialogue with trusted leaders, I am convicted that the American church remains the primary source of failure regarding national advances for human dignity. Yet there is a political entity that has long claimed interest in defending vulnerable lives in the womb, only to fail decade after decade. Let us now turn our eye to the Republican Party.

CHAPTER 7

FAILURE, PART TWO: HOW THE REPUBLICAN PARTY CONTINUES TO ACHIEVE IT

To be very clear, the American church and the Republican Party are *not* the same. Not even close. While I have chosen to discuss the failures of both in these two chapters, they are clearly separate entities. I do not want anyone to proceed from this point with the impression that I am equating them—I am not, unless you consider the fact that they both have failed on this issue.

The Republican platform has, for many years, discussed respect for life, respect for the consciences of health care workers, and the goal of ending taxpayer funding of abortion. As with all politicians, we need to look at what they *do* and not what they say. That is one thing you can say about the Democratic Party—when they promise to expand abortion rights, they mean what they say. For decades, they have demonstrated a willingness to move heaven and earth to keep those promises. They have effectively quashed opposition to the abortion agenda within their ranks. In the 1960s and 1970s, a significant number of the members of the Democratic Party in the United States House and the United States Senate were pro-life. In the early 90s, of

290 Democrats in the House, almost one hundred were pro-life. By 2010, there were less than forty. Those numbers have now dwindled to near non-existence. In 2016, there were only two Democrats in the Congressional Pro-Life Caucus. In 2016, there was only one Democratic senator with a score of less than 100 from NARAL Pro-Choice America, and only three Democratic senators had lifetime scores of less than 100 from the Planned Parenthood Action Fund.[19]

The death blow to pro-life Democrats was the passage of the Affordable Care Act (ACA). Congressman Bart Stupak, D-Minn., was the leader of the pro-life caucus in the Democratic Party in the House, and they were holdouts on voting for the ACA. He was summoned to the White House to meet with President Barack Obama, who verbally promised him that the ACA would never fund abortion—in order to secure the votes of moderate Democrats. The ACA would not have passed in the House without the votes of the Democratic members of their pro-life caucus. During the lead up to the final vote on the ACA, sixty-four Democrats in the House voted for provisions that would have prevented the ACA from funding abortions or subsidizing plans that would cover abortion.[20]

Those Democrats, after having been promised by President Obama that their concerns for life would be respected, then gave Speaker Pelosi their votes and the ACA became law. The Democratic leadership then proceeded with their plans to expand abortion coverage, despite their quiet promises to their own members. Now, only two pro-life Democrats remain in the House. Recently, the co-chair of the Congressional Progressive Caucus, Representative Pramila Jayapal, D-Wash., said in a press conference, "You can't say you're a Democrat…if you're against abortion." She went on to say, "We have to look at all these issues and think about what it means to be a Democrat." She has received support from NARAL for supporting a version of Medicare-for-all that eliminates the Hyde Amendment, a longstanding policy created with bipartisan agreement that blocks direct federal funding for most abortion cases. She has called for primary challenges against Democratic incumbents that are not on board with the most extreme abortion agenda in American history.[21] The Democrats are willing to achieve their agenda for abortion, no matter what it takes—even when it compromises long-term members of their own party. The Republicans, on the other hand....

Republicans who claim to be pro-life simply cannot be believed. For many of them, being pro-life is nothing more than a bullet point on a campaign website! Those who support candidates for public office simply because they claim to be pro-life are just as much a part of the problem as those spineless suits. These incumbent Republicans have records... if voters would only take the time to review them and have a bit of discernment before they go into the voting booth. The pro-life achievements of Republicans in Congress and in statehouses across the country are far more important to consider than their claims to be pro-life. While there are some in elected positions who really take the pro-life position seriously, and I am thankful for them, I have grown weary of those who proclaim their pro-life bona fides but lack the courage to actually do anything meaningful. I am especially wary of those who act as if the pro-life agenda is their top priority but who actually take active actions, usually behind the scenes, to undermine the pro-life movement. There are plenty of elected figures who fall into that category. Then there are lobbying groups that function as nonprofits and raise money on the issue but never do anything meaningful. Some even actively work against strong pro-life legislative efforts. I am about to name a few names and call people out.

Let us start at the top. Mitch McConnell is the current Majority Leader in the United States Senate. He was first elected to the Senate in 1984 and has been re-elected to the Senate five times since then. In an op-ed published by the *Courier-Journal*, the largest newspaper in his home state of Kentucky, McConnell stated on February 22, 2019 that he is a "firm believer in the sanctity of life." While McConnell's voting record does show his support for some anti-abortion actions, his record is notable for its glaring lack of action to defund Planned Parenthood and other abortion providers. During his time as a senator, over 40,000,000 babies have died in abortion clinics. In all that time, there has been not one successful or seemingly sincere effort to strip the abortion industry of federal dollars. As Majority Leader, he could have commissioned an investigation into the 2015 videos that demonstrated Planned Parenthood's profiteering in the baby body parts trade, but he did not—and thus missed an enormous opportunity to expose the abortion industry for what it really is. Missing the opportunity to capitalize on the public outrage over the sale of baby body parts for profit by abortionists compounds his failures on this issue.

Paul Ryan, the recently retired Speaker of the House, is no different. He ran for his seat in the House of Representatives ten times, winning each time. He was always clear about his pro-life convictions. Like McConnell, he had many opportunities to act against the institution of abortion, but he did not. He acted to move countless spending bills forward that always contained the funding demanded by Planned Parenthood and its supporters. The government has been "shut down" when the two parties have reached an impasse multiple times on multiple other issues… but it has never been shut down over the funding that keeps Planned Parenthood's abortion infrastructure open for business. His time in the House prior to becoming Speaker was always spent on committees that handled finances, but he never used that power to affect abortion spending. Then, as Speaker, he had the authority to set the agenda—yet abortion never seemed to be on his radar.

More than 22,000,000 babies died in America's abortion clinics while Paul Ryan served in the House. Actions speak louder than words, and Ryan's words about his pro-life convictions fall flat when his lack of action on pro-life issues is considered.

These are only two names of many on the federal level that deserve recrimination for the inconsistencies in their stated convictions and their records. There are also many on the local level, and I will limit my discussion here to actions by my fellow Tennesseans. I will start with former Congresswoman Diane Black, who left the House in 2018 to run, unsuccessfully, in the Republican gubernatorial race in Tennessee. She never missed an opportunity to point out that she was a former nurse and that she is pro-life. I don't doubt that she does believe that life is worth protecting, and that abortion on demand is wrong. I do believe, however, that she and others like her do not have it nearly as high on their priority lists as they say they do. Congresswoman Black served as the Chair of the Budget Committee in the House, and also served on the Ways and Means Committee—both of which are financial committees. During her time, she ultimately took many actions to authorize spending that included Planned Parenthood's half a billion dollars annually. In a glaring act of inconsistency, she once nearly simultaneously voted to advance a continuing resolution that funded Planned Parenthood while authoring stand-alone legislation that would have defunded Planned Parenthood.

Diane Black is a smart woman. She knew that her stand-alone bill would never have defeated a Senate filibuster… and, even if it did, it never would have been signed into law by President Obama. It was a show bill, one that made the news and padded her pro-life bona fides, but never was going to make a difference. The bill that could have made the difference was the one she voted for—the actual spending bill that continued to fund

Planned Parenthood. We have far too many pro-life legislators who are eager to create a show but are unwilling to draw a real line in the sand and say "No More." They tell us that we just do not understand how Washington works. Oh, I understand how it works. What I do not understand is how people like this, who claim to have such strong pro-life convictions, sleep at night given their lack of effort on the part of the unborn.

We have the same problem in state legislatures, and Tennessee sadly leads the pack on this infamous pattern of practice. At the beginning of the 2019 legislative session, the Tennessee General Assembly convened, and a member of the House introduced, what came to be known as the Heartbeat Bill. The House version of the bill moved quickly through the Health Committee, but because of a variety of competing opinions, influence from a lobbying organization that claims to be pro-life, and an unwillingness to accept knowledgeable input, the House version was, quite frankly, a very bad bill. It was not a bill that would have survived any challenge in court, as it lacked anything that would have made it different or stronger than heartbeat bills that had already been struck down by various federal courts. Constitutional scholars have explained that in order for a case to be accepted for consideration before the Supreme Court, it must be very specific in terms of its legislative intent and have accurate factual information from which conclusions may be drawn. Importantly, it must also have constitutional arguments to consider that have not already been considered and struck down. In other words, a law on abortion must present legitimate medical science coupled with constitutional issues that force the court to reconsider what has previously been ruled upon.

SCOTUS has shown a willingness to reconsider its own opinions on abortion when presented with this kind of law. Nebraska passed a law banning partial-birth abortion, also referred to as intact dilation and extraction.

This is the process by which labor is induced, and when the woman is sufficiently dilated, the abortionist pushes the head up and flips the baby around in order to grab the feet and draw the baby out feet first until only the head remains inside the woman's body. Then, in one final step intended to ensure that the baby is dead before he or she can take a first breath, a sharp instrument is stabbed into the base of the skull from the back of the neck. A suction instrument is then inserted into the hole and the child's brain is suctioned out, allowing the head to collapse and the baby to be more easily delivered in a most certainly dead state. Nebraska's law, while noble, was challenged by notorious late term abortionist Leroy Carhart. In the 2000 decision *Stenberg v. Carhart*, SCOTUS found Nebraska's law unconstitutional when viewed through the lens of *Roe* and *Casey*. They considered in their ruling the fact that the Nebraska law did not include a health exception.

Congress did happen, later, to get this particular issue correct. They passed the federal Partial-Birth Abortion Ban, and in the law, they included specific medical language and used it to craft the legislative intent. They specifically made the case that this particular procedure is never necessary to protect the life or health of the mother, and that there are alternatives to its brutality. Dr. Carhart, again, challenged the law, and the Eighth Circuit Federal Court of Appeals ruled in his favor. U.S. Attorney General Alberto Gonzalez appealed that decision. In 2007, SCOTUS ruled in *Gonzalez v. Carhart* that the federal ban should be upheld, even though it included no exception for the health of the mother. This was a significant reversal of *Stenburg v. Carhart*, and the way in which this was accomplished should be considered when crafting any pro-life legislation.

Fast forward to 2019. The members of the Tennessee House of Representatives who put this bill forward were privately offered this perspective.

They were offered all the medical basis needed to justify consideration of the personhood of the unborn child essentially from conception—even prior to the detection of a visible heartbeat. I was there. My good friend, former Tennessee state representative Joe Carr, and I had worked together for literally hundreds of hours to assemble the medical facts supporting the legislative intent, and had obtained assistance from multiple attorneys to cover the legal and judicial considerations. Mr. Carr is an expert in drafting strong legislation. His work while in the General Assembly resulted in Tennessee having the strongest immigration laws in the country—laws which have never been challenged in court. He brought even more passion and drive to this issue. They declined to consider what was given to them, and the resulting bill was so bad and flawed that it played into the hands of forces that opposed any heartbeat legislation.

Initially, Randy McNally, the Republican Speaker of the Senate (and also the Lieutenant Governor) had instructed the Judiciary Committee Chairman to refuse to hear the House version of the bill in committee because it was so bad. Chairman Bell, also known to be a pro-life Republican, initially complied. Then the Senate sponsor of the bill, Senator Mark Pody, welcomed the medical input and the legislative wisdom offered by me and Carr, a retired member of the House, and the legal opinions of David Fowler, another former legislator who is also a constitutional attorney. He crafted an amendment to the House bill that addressed the issues. Speaker McNally's opposition did not abate at this point. It increased. The opposition was bolstered by the actions of Tennessee Right to Life. Tennessee Right to Life and its head, Brian Harris, did good work in getting a Tennessee constitutional amendment on abortion passed in 2014. They have defended the ability of Tennesseans to have "Choose Life" license plates on their vehicles and have donated some funds to Tennessee crisis pregnancy centers.

However, Tennessee Right to Life (RTL) also has a history of inexplicably opposing good legislative efforts. Pro-life members of the General Assembly crave the endorsement of RTL and have done RTL's bidding. TN RTL endorsed what was known as a Trigger Bill, which ultimately passed during this session. This piece of legislation, of which RTL is very proud, does nothing to advance the pro-life cause. The Trigger Bill will only be an achievement if someone else is successful in challenging *Roe*, and in that event would restore Tennessee law to what it was prior to *Roe*. Additionally, if efforts to pass a federal constitutional amendment overturning *Roe* were ever successful, the same end would be achieved. This law made the news but won't make a difference unless someone else fights and wins.

Simultaneous to their efforts to pass this bill, they openly opposed the Heartbeat Bill. Their talking points, which had remarkable similarities to Planned Parenthood's press releases about this bill, were parroted by Republicans in the state Senate. (Interestingly, Planned Parenthood chose to expend no effort on opposing the Trigger Bill.) They published their opposition talking points on the RTL webpage on March 5, 2019, weeks before the text of Senator Pody's amendment was available for them to consider. They were invited to assist and contribute to the crafting of the bill, and they declined—repeatedly. Their final response to Senator Pody was revelatory. It appears that the TN RTL leadership does not believe that *Roe* can be overturned.

I was involved in a private meeting scheduled by Senator Pody. He asked me and David Fowler, the president of Family Action Council Tennessee, to attend with him. Mr. Fowler was once in the state Senate; he is a constitutional attorney and has been a pro-life activist for decades. He helped craft the legal arguments to consider and make a part of this bill. Senator Pody took us with him and another truly pro-life senator, Janice Bowling, to the office of the Lieutenant Governor. Tennessee Attorney General Herb Slattery was also in attendance. They both had voiced public opposition to the bill on the grounds that it was "constitutionally suspect." They claimed that the risk of being challenged and failing—and then being held responsible for the victor's legal fees—was an irresponsible risk of state funds. Note that their rhetoric reveals a highly disingenuous position. In Tennessee, we currently have a record-breaking fiscal surplus. These same senators in this same legislative session have worked hard to pass other pieces of legislation which will be challenged, such as a bill for some educational reform. But they did not have those fiscal concerns in mind on issues they wished to pass.

We met with them with the good faith intent to persuade them to work with us, to help make the bill stronger and to their liking. We were not well-received. Lt. Governor McNally was reluctant to even shake my hand as the meeting started. Then, as we presented our case, he and Slattery had only oppositional comments and arguments. As we progressed through an hour-long discussion, their arguments diminished. Senator Pody repeatedly asked them to consider what they could do to offer suggestions for improvement, and his respectful requests were met with silence. McNally was visibly angry as we left his office. The Judiciary Committee meeting for which the bill had been placed on the calendar was to be the next day. McNally began calling Republican members of the Judiciary Committee into his office one by one to discuss the matter with them.

The next day, the bill was the twentieth item on the Judiciary Committee's agenda. The nineteenth item was the RTL supported Trigger Bill. When the RTL representative was called to testify to the committee, he opened with the statement: "I am here to testify in support of the Human Life Protection Act, which is the *only* piece of pro-life legislation before this committee tonight which TN RTL supports." He then proceeded to spend approximately the same amount of time attacking the Heartbeat Bill as he did supporting the Trigger Bill. His bill was passed out of committee on a 7-2 vote with no debate at all.

Then the Heartbeat Bill came forth. Senator Pody introduced the proposed legislation, and for almost an hour and a half I gave medical testimony and answered questions. David Fowler presented compelling and novel constitutional considerations, defending our premise that this bill presents the issue in a way not previously considered by SCOTUS. For a moment, I actually thought that we had been successful in persuading the committee to vote affirmatively to send the Heartbeat Bill to the floor of the full Senate for a vote. I was sadly mistaken.

Chairman Bell began reading from a long statement, obviously prepared before he had heard any of the testimony. In it he gave voice to every objection that Senate leadership and RTL had been spouting for weeks. He used that as justification to send the bill to what in the Tennessee General Assembly is known as "Summer Study." Summer Study is almost always a legislative graveyard that is used to put proposed legislation opposed by leadership to a slow and quiet death. The vote to send it to Summer Study was then taken, and five members of the Committee voted to do so, three opposed, and one abstained. Interestingly, the office of the Lt. Governor used social media to release a statement praising the Judiciary Committee's decision to send the bill to Summer Study *several moments before* the vote to do so was taken. His statement was eerily similar to the Chairman's statement on his decision to do so. The fix was in before the hearing was even held.

Senator Pody had two options at that point. One was to accept the Summer Study decision and make the best effort to prepare for a two-day hearing scheduled in August and hope for the best. Senator Pody felt, as did I, that we needed to try every opportunity possible to get this passed before next year. He found, in the Senate rules, an option known as Rule 63. This is an option rarely used in the Tennessee Senate, and it allows a senator to make a motion in an open Senate session to have the Senate vote on whether or not to rescue a bill from the committee system and bring it directly to the full floor of the Senate for debate and a vote. He made his intention to do this clear, as he is an open, transparent, and honest man. He had intended to do so on Thursday, April 18, 2019. He did communicate with Senate leadership and offered them the opportunity to avoid this action if he was allowed to bring it back to the Judiciary Committee for reconsideration and additional debate now, instead of waiting for Summer Study. That is an option that is allowable under Senate rules.

Just before the April 18 session convened, he was approached by the clerk of the Senate and told that it would be allowed to return to committee; he acted in good faith and did not make his Rule 63 motion. Then, at the end of the evening's session, the calendars for the following week were announced and the Senate quickly adjourned—without the Heartbeat Bill having been officially placed back on the Judiciary Committee agenda. He approached the clerk and asked why this happened. The clerk looked him in the face and said, "Sorry, I made a mistake." Understand, "mistakes" like this do not happen. Dirty tricks and lies do, but mistakes do not.

Senator Pody remained resolute. The next Senate session was scheduled to be on Monday, April 22, 2019. He held a press conference beforehand and discussed his intentions openly, with many supporters backing him. He then went into session, and at the proper time respectfully made his motion. Senator Bowling took the floor and spoke eloquently in support of the bill. Three other senators spoke of their opposition to supporting the bill now. They proclaimed their pro-life bona fides and quoted Scripture… and then rationalized their opposition. Then, in a move apparently planned ahead of time, a motion to table Senator Pody's motion for a Rule 63 vote was made, and then quickly seconded. Speaker McNally immediately called for a voice vote and ignored Senator Pody's proper request for a recorded vote. The motion to table the vote passed on a voice vote less than sixty seconds after it was made; there is no record of which senators voted to table the vote, because they fear accountability with their districts.

The Democrats and Planned Parenthood did not have to lift a finger or spend a dime to defeat efforts to get this bill signed into law. The Republicans and Tennessee Right to Life did their work for them. They were enabled by the silence from the pulpits of the churches many legislators attend…and by the ignorance of voters who continue to elect officials who say one thing and do another on important issues.

After the dust settled a bit, I was contacted via email by Paul Linton, an attorney who works with TN Right to Life. He asked me to help clarify his understanding of the concept of viability as I discussed it in the Senate Judiciary Committee hearing, and he asked for help locating the specific medical references I had used. I responded respectfully but firmly with the following text in an email:

Mr. Linton,

I offer my apology for taking so long to respond, and I am glad to have heard from you. This issue is obviously one of critical importance. I am hopeful that we can work together in good faith, but you must understand that I feel it necessary to inquire as to your motivations. I feel that it would have been more appropriate for you and TN Right to Life to have reached out to us before testimony was given, but not only did that not occur, multiple efforts by Senator Pody to enlist RTL's assistance or even consideration were ignored. If the goal is to work together to achieve something meaningful then I will be happy to spend the time working with you in any way as we move towards the Summer Study session which has now been scheduled. If, however, RTL simply wishes to bolster their opposition to this proposed legislation, I will have to decline.

I await your response.

Most sincerely yours,

C. Brent Boles, MD

His response, sadly predictable given the RTL behavior in the lead-up to the recent legislative session, was to reaffirm his belief that such a bill has no chance of being heard by the Supreme Court. I must confess that I fail to understand why those who have chosen to oppose legislation like this rely on statements that this bill is "unconstitutional" or is "constitutionally suspect" as their rationalization for opposing it. Of course it is unconstitutional and constitutionally suspect! It must be in conflict with that which is considered constitutional under current judicial precedent in order to make a difference! It is rather insulting to me that these people think that a statement like that is supposed to put all discussion to bed. Here is the proper perspective for anyone who wishes to see *Roe* and its obscene descendants overturned: That which is currently "constitutional" is only considered to be such when viewed through the lens of *Roe* and its bastard descendants. Anything that will ever achieve a change in what is currently considered to be constitutional must begin as something that is patently and boldly unconstitutional when evaluated in view of *Roe*.

Half-measures and incrementalism will not succeed. Because some may take this statement as disparaging their work, let me explain my perspective on this briefly. I fully support states that have passed such pro-life policies as informed consent laws, clinic safety regulations, and waiting period laws. These are important policies to protect women's health that have a strong basis in medical ethics. Such baseline laws also serve to save some vulnerable lives in the womb, though will not win the war against *Roe*. In some liberal-majority states, and sometimes at the federal level, incremental policies are the only ones that have a possibility of being enacted. However, in a state like Tennessee, with a Governor and both legislative chambers claiming to be pro-life, such small steps are inadequate. Failing to advance bold challenges to *Roe v. Wade* and other established judicial precedents reveals a lack of commitment to the pro-life cause of saving as many lives as possible, by any means possible. We are in this to win and ultimately abolish abortion, not perpetuate "pro-life" fundraising and political campaigns.

Today, the driving judicial precedent states that the individual's right to terminate a pregnancy is superior to the unborn child's right to life itself. Thus, any measure that does not bring that child's rights to the forefront of the discussion, with conclusive proof of the living status of the human unborn person whose life is at stake, will fail. You would think that such a conclusion is simple, but apparently it is not. I am a trained medical diagnostician; when I see a problem, I naturally consider what issues have created the problem. In order to determine what issues are at fault, you must examine things carefully and sometimes conduct testing. Then, once you understand the "why," you can make progress toward a treatment. Understanding "why" a problem exists is crucial to the process of achieving a remedy. In this case, there are only a limited number of explanations as to "why" there is opposition from supposedly pro-life legislators, attorneys, and organizations.

Some have said that they want such legislation to be as strong as possible in order to have the greatest chance of judicial success. There is a simple test which allows us to determine the truth of such a statement and it is this: work with us to make the legislation better. If those who made statements such as this are truly sincere, then they would get on board and work with us. As we approach Summer Study, I will give those individuals the benefit of the doubt and see if they put their money where their mouth is.

There are a limited number of reasonable explanations for the behavior of those who maintain a steadfast opposition to real efforts to overturn *Roe*.

- They do not believe it can be done—in which case they should demonstrate integrity and stop their efforts in this struggle. Walking away would clear the stage for those who are willing to fight.

- They believe in a less aggressive approach—an incrementalism, if you will—which has historically enjoyed little success and proven inadequate to challenge the pro-choice status quo. They fail to see that, as such, it is an unwise approach that should be abandoned in most contexts.

- They may truly believe in their hearts that they are pro-life, but the issue for them takes a backseat to other issues—such as being unwilling to risk state funds to defend meaningful legislation in court. Those who claim to believe in the sanctity of life and the need to protect unborn life, and who campaign as if it is an issue of prime importance, must step up to the plate and act as if their words are true.

- They are not truly pro-life at all and realize that in order to win elections in their districts they must pretend to be, or risk losing their elections. These are the people for whom being pro-life is simply a bullet point on a campaign website, or a statement in a campaign speech.

At the time of this writing, our hope is now fixed on Summer Study, and we will complete our good faith effort and work to do everything possible to persuade the General Assembly that this is a fight worth having. I can only hope that those who are truly pro-life will elevate the issue to a place of first and utmost importance as we move forward.

CHAPTER 8

GOD WANTS TO ANSWER OUR PRAYERS TO END ABORTION

I want to share a story with you. Years ago, a patient came into my office, and we had the most inspiring conversation. She gave me permission to share her story; I will refer to her as Jane, although that is not her real name. This story is told to you exactly as she relayed it to me. It carries the unmistakable ring of truth, because the evidence of her changed life testifies to the truth.

Jane shared with me that she has now had control over her drug addiction for several years. Her problem began through no fault of her own. She had been in an accident, then was on chronic narcotic pain medication for an extended period of time. Once completely healed and no longer in need of the narcotics for pain, she had a physiological need for them—an addiction. She began to use whatever she could get her hands on; it didn't matter what it was. It branched out from narcotics into other substances like cocaine. Her life was a mess. She already had two children. One day, she began to suspect that she was pregnant once again and a feeling of absolute horror came upon her. She knew that all the substances she had been putting into her body would have been horrible for the baby. She knew that she would have an exceedingly difficult time living with the guilt if her baby had birth defects and developmental disabilities as a result of her choices. So she decided to have an abortion.

Her mother and stepfather did their best to talk her out of doing that. She had no money, and was able to persuade her sister to give her two thousand dollars and take her to an abortion clinic in Nashville. She walked in the door confused, sad, and terrified. Her sister waited in the car for her.

Now, you must understand something about abortion clinics. Their business is abortion—it puts cash in their pockets and keeps the gates of hell (their front doors) open. They never refer to the baby as a baby. They never say anything or do anything to help the woman feel connected to the baby. In her 2004 diatribe *The War On Choice*, former Planned Parenthood president Gloria Feldt never once refers to the baby as a baby. Their recent president, Cecile Richards, has repeatedly said that the question of when life begins "isn't relevant to the conversation" about abortion. They know that if a woman feels a connection to the baby, she is far less likely to abort. They know that once a woman sees a picture of the baby moving around on ultrasound and hears the heartbeat, then she is more than 90 percent likely to walk out the door without an abortion. As a result, abortion clinic ultrasound technicians never let the woman see the screen. They never refer to the baby as a baby. They never personalize the pregnancy for the woman, because that doesn't get them paid.

Keep those facts in mind as you read what happened next. Jane was having her ultrasound done. The technician began talking to her about the baby, saying things like "Oh, what a strong, healthy heartbeat" and "Everything looks normal" and "These are great pictures" and—the biggest no-no for an abortion clinic ultrasound technician—"It's a boy!" Jane was upset.

She couldn't believe that her "choice" was becoming more and more difficult. She wondered why things were happening the way they were. The
ultrasound was finally complete, and her next stop was a conversation with
the "doctor" that was there that day to kill babies for cash.

Jane sat across the desk from the man tasked with performing her abortion. He looked down at her file, looked at the ultrasound report, and began to look distinctly uncomfortable. He even began to sweat. He fidget-
ed around in his seat. He then did something that abortion clinic doctors
simply do not ever do. He closed her file, and said, "I don't know why I am
doing this, but I am not going to do this procedure for you." Jane asked why
and he responded with: "I do not know. But I am not going to do it." He
then wrote down the name of another facility and told her that if she really
wanted it done, then she could go there. Then he ended the conversation
and dismissed her.

Jane left the abortion facility upset and confused. She didn't know what
to do. It was not that she wanted to have the abortion—but she wanted to
have a baby with potentially diminished abilities even less. She didn't want
to spend the rest of her life looking at the consequences of her behavior. She
told her sister what had happened, and they left to drive home.

As they drove home, they called their mother. Of course, their mother
was overcome with relief. She put their stepfather on the phone. When Jane
told him the story, he broke down. He said, "Do you know what I have been
doing? For the last three hours, I have been laying on the floor crying and
praying that God would have someone there at that place talk you out of it.
I have been praying that the doctor would refuse to do it." Let that sink in
for a moment....

Jane got serious about getting help for her addiction. She became clean,
quit using harmful drugs, and hasn't used since then. A few months later,

she delivered a healthy baby boy with no disabilities and no problems. He did not experience withdrawal. He is now a few years old, a very special little boy who has exceeded all his developmental milestones.

Jane now attends meetings, like most former addicts do. She no longer struggles with the cravings for the drugs, but still goes to the meetings because she wants to help others. God is honoring her efforts and her desires to help others. Every week she is able to be an inspirational story to someone and a testimony to the power of God. She told me that there is never a single week that goes by when she is not able to help at least one addict. Because God responded to intense prayer, not only was her baby saved, her life was transformed; and now that blessing of transformation flows into the lives of others on a regular basis. God wants to honor the prayers of His people on the issue of abortion. Make the scourge of abortion in our land a daily prayer point and grow your prayer life on this topic. God will honor your efforts, just like He honored the efforts of Jane's stepfather.

Did you see the recent movie *Unplanned*? If you did not, you must find a way to see it. It is the true story of Abby Johnson as told in her book, also named *Unplanned*. Abby made Planned Parenthood history by becoming the youngest person to ever be a Planned Parenthood abortion clinic director. During the time that she worked for them at a clinic in Texas, more than twenty-two thousand abortions were performed there, either surgically or medically. She began to have reservations about Planned Parenthood's business model becoming more aggressive in its goal of profiting from abortion. Then, one day she was called in to assist with the ultrasound portion of an ultrasound-guided abortion. Seeing what she then saw was the tipping point for her, and she quickly left the organization. She was taken to court by Planned Parenthood, but was victorious. Now her story is changing hearts and minds in America on this issue.

Before her dramatic exit from the abortion industry, there were those who were praying for Abby. The movie depicts the difficulty her parents had with her choice to work for Planned Parenthood, as they were pro-life. It also clearly shows that her husband was not a fan of her occupational choice, and it shows that they had been praying for her persistently for years. Then there is the character of Shawn Carney, who co-founded the national movement 40 Days for Life with Catholic pro-life educator David Bereit. With a small team of women and men, they began praying on the sidewalk outside of Johnson's Planned Parenthood facility in the fall of 2004. It is now a national movement that has people praying outside of abortion clinics all over the country. Standing peacefully outside of abortion clinics, they pray for children, mothers, and the workers. There are now hundreds of thousands of volunteer intercessors who participate in this effort. In a recent interview with *The Christian Post*, Carney credits faithful prayer as having had a powerful role in what happened in Abby's life and what is now happening in the pro-life movement.[22] He was asked by the interviewer: "How have you seen continuous, unbroken prayer, the kind of intercession you all practice outside abortion clinics, dismantle the evil in the spiritual realm?" He responded, "It's just the timeless battle of life versus death. And Christ is the victor…There is so much spiritual warfare. And the devil certainly works through abortion to disguise himself and to convince people that it's a responsible thing, a good thing. That it's health care and that it's wonderful. And yet, it's something that, when you step back…we wouldn't wish this on members of ISIS. We wouldn't wish this on our greatest enemy."

Prayers to end abortion are working. In one scene in the film, Abby tells Shawn that even Planned Parenthood knows that prayer makes a difference. She referred to it as a "dirty little secret" at Planned Parenthood, which tracks statistics of appointments kept and appointments missed. Johnson states that the rate of women scheduled for abortions who do not come to their appointments skyrockets on days when people are praying peacefully outside the clinics. Prayer works.

Post-abortive people need prayer. It is a little-known fact that one of every four women attending American churches each Sunday has had an abortion. Many times, the fathers of aborted children are in church as well. They are virtually all in pain, and usually have no idea how to begin to move forward and away from that pain and toward healing and wholeness. If your church has an organized ministry that works to meet the needs of post-abortive people, then get on board with it and be trained to assist. Pray for that ministry regularly. And if your church does not have such a ministry, then begin gathering regularly with a group of like-minded people. Begin praying for an opportunity to develop a ministry through which the needs of post-abortive people can be met.

One of the most successful ministries I have ever seen is a prison ministry, which did not exist ten years ago. The need for it was passionately on the heart of a friend who is a pastor, John Spurgeon Ponukamati. He and his wife, along with me and my wife and one other couple, began meeting one evening each week. For almost a year, we prayed regularly for the things that were on our minds, and the birth of a prison ministry was always on the prayer list. That ministry now has led to the conversions and baptisms of literally hundreds of inmates. They have reached out to the families of those incarcerated, ministering to them and their children as well. The superintendent of the correctional facility began tracking recidivism rates among those released inmates who were a part of the program; the rate of recidivism was dramatically reduced. Lives were changed, and people were brought into the kingdom. Lives were lifted out of despair because of a beginning rooted in dedicated, sustained, faithful prayer—and God's response to that.

Being post-abortive can be like being in a prison in your own mind. There is despair and loss. It can dominate your every thought and every action. Sometimes, because the pain is too great, other issues develop—relationship dysfunction and substance abuse to dull the pain are common occurrences. The post-abortive individual may need ministry as much as the inmate or the inmate's family. The similarities between these issues are striking, and both are issues that are important to the heart of our God. In Matthew 25, Jesus says, "Come, you who are blessed by my Father; take your inheritance, the kingdom prepared for you since the creation of the world. For I was hungry and you gave me something to eat, I was thirsty and you gave me something to drink, I was a stranger and you invited me in, I needed clothes and you clothed me, I was sick and you looked after me, I was in prison and you came to visit me" (Matthew 25:34-36, NIV). Post-abortive people are hungry and thirsty for mercy, healing, and compassion—and often they have no idea where to find it. They are often sick in ways that cannot be clearly seen, and are in prisons of pain in their own minds; they can find no release or escape. They need God's love and forgiveness to be ministered to them. Once set free, they can often become the most ardent and vigorous serving members of any church or ministry. Successful ministry is birthed in and maintained by vigilant, persistent prayer—so pray and then watch God move.

A young woman named Natalie Brumfield in Birmingham, Alabama has faithfully carried out the call of God on her life through pro-life prayer. Over the past decade, she and her husband, Matthew, have organized local prayer groups for 40 Days for Life and Bound4LIFE International. They are parents of four children, including three adopted. When asked about why to pray in such difficult environments, she answers that it's because God asked us to. "It is not easy to constantly pray at abortion centers," she wrote in *The Christian Post*.[23] "After many years, it's heavy on me. It's grueling. It doesn't make me popular. I've lost special friends over the years. And the reality of what goes on inside the buildings rips my heart open over and over again."

She continues: "But it isn't about me. It's about that single woman who has no one to turn to and feels absolutely hopeless. It's about that baby who may not live to see the world outside of her/his mommy's tummy. It's about being there for others and helping to carry their pain." She cites Philippians 2:3-4: "Rather, in humility, value others above yourselves, not looking to your own interests but each of you to the interests of the others."

Pastor Allen Jackson, senior pastor of World Outreach Church in Murfreesboro, Tennessee, discussed the issue of abortion in a recent sermon. His perspective was very well stated, and his message was well received by those who heard it. Pastor Allen is well-known for devoting time in his teaching to the topic of prayer, and this message included prayer as part of a proper response by the church to the issue of abortion. At the conclusion of the message, he offered two prayers which were prayed together by all those who were present. I have included them here.

The first prayer is for those who have been involved in abortion in any way:

Lord Jesus Christ—I believe You are the Son of God and the only way to God, that You died on the cross for my sins and rose again from the dead. I confess my sin before You, the sin of abortion and any participation in facilitating or encouraging abortion. I know that You are the creator of life, and I have sinned against You. I receive Your forgiveness now. I choose to forgive myself. I also forgive any other person/persons involved. I ask You now to break the curse of this sin, and I invite Your blessing upon my life. In Jesus' name, amen.

The second prayer is to be offered by the church corporately:

Lord Jesus, we come to You in repentance for the sins of our nation; we have turned our backs upon You. We have been in rebellion to Your commandments, specifically "You Shall Not Murder." We have not treated life as sacred, and we are grieved by our sin. For the sake of convenience and pursuit of our selfish interests, we have ignored You. Through complacency and silence, we have been complicit in this sin; we are guilty. For this we humbly ask You to forgive us, forgive our nation, and awaken Your Church. Therefore, O God, we cry out to You, HAVE MERCY on us. We believe Your Word is true—that if Your people who are called by Your name humble themselves and pray, that You will hear our prayer and bring healing to our land. In Jesus' name, amen.

CHAPTER 9

A WINNING STRATEGY

The battle for life must be waged on a number of fronts. It must be fought in an unflinching and uncompromising way. The other side will never compromise—that much is very clear. They have abandoned their old deceptive adage of "safe, legal, and rare." They have unrelentingly pressed the judicial advantages given to them by SCOTUS precedent, to the point that we are now actually having to debate if a baby who survives an abortion has any rights whatsoever. Their definition of when a person is a person deserving of rights has shifted—ours cannot and must not. There is only one defensible and science-based position: that life begins at conception. Choosing any point other than conception to grant a person the actual rights of personhood would be an arbitrary choice, subject to later changes of whim and political expediency. That is neither moral nor ethical, neither right nor defensible.

The Supreme Court thought that it found a way out of having to rule on competing rights and interests by ignoring the personhood of the unborn child. Their misguided majority opinion in *Roe v. Wade* inevitably has led to an avalanche of judicial decisions that do not make sense. SCOTUS has perpetuated the injustices of *Roe*, and has created a class of *untermensch* (to use a horrific term from the Holocaust) that are considered disposable simply because they are unwanted or inconvenient. A multi-billion-dollar annual business of death has evolved, with power and influence over politics, medicine, and other sectors of our nation.

In his fifth century B.C. work, *The Art of War*, Chinese military genius Sun Tzu penned thirteen chapters on military strategy, tactics, and weaponry. It has been considered a classic work for battlefield leaders and commanders for more than two thousand years. A review of the summaries of each of the thirteen chapters makes one thing clear—Tzu's teaching focused on knowledge, understanding, and the importance of being well-informed. He makes it clear that wisdom and knowledge are far more important than the size of the military force or the exact nature of the weaponry carried into battle. He focuses on how even knowledge of the terrain is critical to victory...and that defeat is almost certain for the uninformed and poorly prepared warrior.

How does this translate into something applicable in our battle for life? That should be clear to all by now. Those of us who choose to engage in this must equip *ourselves* and *those around us* with knowledge, wisdom, and a thorough understanding of the issues. We must know the truth so completely that we are able to respond quickly, forcefully, and accurately when those on the other side speak that which is inaccurate, or misleading, or simply not true. In an earlier chapter, I quoted an important principle found in the Old Testament book of Hosea—that we perish for a lack of knowledge. In the case of abortion, babies perish for our lack of knowledge.

Educating ourselves and others is only the beginning. It is of critical importance—indeed, it is foundational and without it we will not ultimately succeed. It is, however, only the beginning. There are a number of things that must flow from being prepared and practiced in the art of pro-life apologetics.

We must care enough to be activists on this subject. This does not mean that we must devote ourselves to the full-time work of defending life. While that has been and will be the vocational choice made by some, it will not be for most. There is so much that can be done at any of several levels by anyone who wishes to devote even a modest amount of time or resources to our struggle. You can volunteer at a local crisis pregnancy center. There are thousands of them across the country, and the vast majority of Americans will find themselves within an hour's drive of at least one center. These nonprofit centers survive because of the financial generosity of supporters and the time given by volunteers. They make an immeasurable difference in hundreds of thousands of lives. They not only support women who have found themselves in difficult and unexpected situations; they also serve as community for those of us who call ourselves pro-life. That community raises awareness, educates, makes opportunities more clearly and easily accessible, and gives us confidence. When we see the successes in the lives of people to whom we have ministered, we naturally become more confident in the rightness of our cause and our abilities to make a difference.

There will, inevitably, be those who wish that they could be involved, and who wish that they could make a difference. But they are, themselves, post-abortive and cannot conceive of being able to get involved and make a difference; or they may feel that they are simply unworthy because of their past decisions. Nothing could be further from the truth! In fact, some of the most effective activism comes from people who have abortion as part of their story. If this is speaking to you, then please listen. Consider the truth that having your past as prologue may be exactly what motivates you to be effective and may be that which will give you credibility when you speak to this subject. Your story matters. Do not discount your own ability to make a difference in the here and now as well as the future, because of what happened back then.

Other opportunities for activism are relatively easy to find. There are those who feel called to be present on the very front lines and wish to join those who pray outside of abortion clinics. These people will be there to pray and to be available to speak to women who have chosen to visit such a place because they are either considering abortion or have decided to proceed with an abortion. Many churches will have a group of members who participate in this process. The training and equipping which occurs for those people will be highly variable based on the church and on the target locations. If your church is one of these which has chosen to take part in this battle, then seek out what your church has to offer. If your church does not have an organized sidewalk advocacy program, I will make you aware of two programs that should be easily accessible to most people who are interested, both of which have a national presence.

Sidewalk Advocates for Life (www.sidewalkadvocates.org) is an organization that trains and equips people to be on the front lines, preparing them to be kind and life-affirming. I admire their innovative and strategic techniques for reaching people and making a difference. On their website, you can access information to get started with their well-designed training program. As discussed previously, many times the most effective activists are those for whom abortion is part of their story. I am aware of one individual who had not truly dealt with the impact her abortion had on her life until she took advantage of the opportunity to receive post-abortive ministry through a *Surrendering The Secret* group. As she progressed through this study, she gained the boldness to get her church involved and active on the front lines of this issue. Now her church has become a training site for Sidewalk Advocates for Life. Because of her own abortion, she became an activist and now is having a tremendous impact in the equipping and training of people who may have wanted to be involved for a long time but just did not know how. Being a forerunner isn't always easy, but it will always have an impact.

40 Days For Life is another organization that is active across America, and which has an international presence. If you saw the movie *Unplanned*, the local group Coalition for Life that played a key role in the life of Abby Johnson has now morphed into the national coalition 40 Days for Life. Their website (www.40daysforlife.com) will inform you as to what opportunities there are within the proven success of their framework. Stories like the life of Abby Johnson show us all the potential of giving our time to being a kind, truthful, and steadfast presence outside of abortion clinics. We never know when that one person may have their mind and their heart changed and then go on to have a huge impact. While I have devoted time and space in this chapter to just these two, please know that this list is not exhaustive by any means. Other worthy and worthwhile groups exist and are accessible to many. Save the Storks (www.savethestorks.com) is one such group, and it's worth looking into what they do and how you can become involved. My wife and I became aware of this particular organization when we met their staff member Victoria Robinson. She was helping to prepare, on a grassroots level, for the release of the recent movie *Unplanned*. Because of social media exposure, she invited us to a private pre-release screening of *Unplanned* where we were able to meet the producer of the movie and the lead actress, Ashley Bratcher. When we attended the screening a month before the general release of the film, it awakened in us both a sense of urgency to do more. Victoria is active on a national level with Save the Storks, which plays a vital role in coming alongside pregnancy centers and enabling them to be more effective in their local communities. Victoria's passion for the issue of life arose in part because of her own abortion story. An accomplished author, her book *They*

Lied To Us (written under the name Victoria Koloff) is a compilation of stories from women who are post-abortive.

Activism can, and must, take on more roles than the ones discussed thus far. Some local, state, and national pro-life advocates are deeply involved in child welfare. The pro-life movement needs to become more educated and engaged regarding ways to protect vulnerable children *after* birth. The U.S. child welfare system involves a complex web of adoption agencies, social workers, sacrificial foster care households, and a host of nonprofit groups seeking to help children. When a new birth mother decides to allow another couple to adopt her child, or when evidence comes to light of a parent's abuse or addiction, these entities get involved as empowered by state laws. To begin to understand this system and its many opportunities—including the need for adoptive and foster parents—advocates could begin with Christian Alliance For Orphans (www.cafo.org). This coalition group offers a myriad of resources, current statistics, and access to a network of well-established adoption and foster care groups. With government and private entities working in tandem, child welfare brings us to the political and legislative front.

Make no mistake, state and federal lawmaking is another front line in the battle for life. The American voter has historically been a sleeping giant, and it is past time for the pro-life voting giant to awaken from a long slumber. Politicians most often will only respond to pressure, or to rewards. Those on the Left who support abortion at all times, for any reason, do so not necessarily because they really believe that life doesn't begin at conception or that the unborn really isn't a person. Rather, they support it because they fear losing the votes of abortion supporters, and they wish to maintain the inflow of campaign cash from Planned Parenthood. Many of those on the Right crave the endorsements of pro-life organizations in order to appeal to their voting base, and they have historically not been held accountable for their failure to enact and defend meaningful reforms once in office. It is time for that to change.

In the book *Personhood: The Tree of Life*, editor Daniel Becker has assembled an excellent strategic body of work that I highly recommend for those interested in a deeper dive into this issue. The book is a compilation of essays from individuals involved with Personhood Alliance, whose mission you can study more fully at www.personhood.org. In the eighteenth chapter, "Political Failure and the Path to Victory," the writer quotes pro-life film producer Jason Scott Jones. I wholeheartedly agree with his concise and succinct strategy.

> We must help our friends, punish our enemies, and avenge ourselves on traitors. And "friends" cannot be defined as "anyone who threw us a rhetorical bone." We shouldn't be "disappointed" when people we supported wilt under pressure and turn against us. We should be enraged, and ready to impose retribution. We should work to destroy such a politician's career, and send him back to practicing small-town law under an assumed name with an unlisted phone number.

As stated by chapter author Christopher Kurka, board member of Personhood Alliance and Alaska Right To Life Executive Director, "One of the main reasons the pro-life movement loses politically is that politicians fear Planned Parenthood's political wrath more than they fear us." While this may all sound overly aggressive, these seemingly hostile stances arise from a very obvious truth: those who campaign as pro-life candidates, but who govern as if life doesn't matter, have, as of yet, not been held accountable for their failures. They have not yet paid a price for the votes they cast. While I reject employing the politics of personal destruction in the pro-life movement, I believe that we will not see meaningful action from legislators and politicians whom we do not hold to account. It is time to remember that they work for us. It is time that we rise up, make our voices heard, and make our convictions count.

If we would make our views and convictions known to all those currently in office, and *followed through* firmly and unflinchingly through two or three elections cycles, then we would see real change. Those who live up to their words—who show that they listen and respond appropriately—would be rewarded by continuing to have our support with campaign donations and with our votes. Those who do not see the light should then feel the heat. We should be aggressively involved with vigorous primary challenges for those whose words and actions fail to demonstrate a satisfactory degree of internal consistency. Convince them to vote as they should for life, or vote them out. Even just one or two examples in each state in one election cycle would send a clear, unmistakable message that the pro-life voting giant is awake and will never again slumber while babies die. Legislators who call themselves "pro-life" would take the mantle of responsibility they carry much more seriously if we, the pro-life voters, begin to behave as if life really matters.

The other side has no problems with a no-holds-barred bare-knuckles strategy within their own ranks. It is clear as Democratic candidates for the 2020 presidential race come forward—their unified position on abortion is abortion-all-the-way-to-the-due-date and infanticide-if-the-unwanted-baby-is-born-alive. There are currently no exceptions to this. The co-chair of the House Progressive Caucus recently made it clear that supporting abortion rights with no restrictions is "what it means to be a Democrat"—and that those unwilling to toe the party line should expect primary challenges. The Left advances because they mean what they say, and they act on it.

We also have an opportunity to affect policy decisions made by lobbying groups such as Right to Life. The example of Tennessee Right to Life and their inexplicable opposition to meaningful pro-life legislation is discussed in more detail in a previous chapter, but they merit mention here as well. TN RTL and organizations like them depend on donations to survive and thrive, and without contributions they would do neither. It is time for them to earn their keep. They can lead, or follow, or get out of the way. Here in Tennessee, it seems apparent that they won't respond to reason, therefore they must begin to feel pressure. If a difference is to be made, pressure must be applied.

The key failing of many who consider themselves to be pro-life activists and legislators, including those in TN RTL and those members of the Tennessee General Assembly who opposed recent efforts to pass heartbeat legislation, is the belief that incrementalism is the proper way to address the issue. This particular view is that it is most appropriate to whittle away at abortion rights, moving slowly and deliberately to advance the cause of life. In this way of thinking, it is felt to be most prudent to take gradual steps to reduce the numbers of abortions—because any bold measures are sure to fail. In some states, or during liberal-majority sessions in Congress, it is reasonable to advance bills that, for instance, protect born-alive abortion survivors. This policy would save relatively few lives compared to all lost nationally to abortion. Yet, it serves to bring clarity to the national debate over life, as it speaks directly to the headlines we are all troubled about regarding legal infanticide. Furthermore, I regard waiting period laws, informed consent laws, and clinic safety standard laws as important measures. Evidence shows that they improve women's health care. However, such policies will never win the war against *Roe v. Wade*.

I contend that the incremental approach taken by many in the pro-life movement since 1973 is fatally flawed. It has failed at almost every turn, while those who support unlimited abortion rights have enjoyed vast success in advancing their agenda. While there have been a few notable successes, such as passage of a federal partial-birth abortion ban and the subsequent victory at the Supreme Court level in *Gonzales v. Carhart*, most incrementally formulated legislation fails. It fails because that which is considered constitutional is deemed to be so by being viewed through the lens of *Roe* and *Casey*. As long as these SCOTUS precedents determine that which is constitutional, incremental legislation will not save babies nor protect women from the predatory nature of the abortion industry—and will almost always fail.

In the journal *First Things*, writer Philip Jefferey posted a column titled "Against Pro-life Incrementalism" which points out several very important considerations.[24] He posits that, "We must escape the defeatist mentality that animates incrementalism. We are not going to make progress if we do not take bold steps forward." He goes on to correctly state that this is a moral issue. In reference to the recent Alabama Heartbeat law, he says that it must be defended "because it clarifies the moral stakes. It insists that the question at hand is not about week-cutoffs, exceptions, and the marginal cases that dominate debate, but about whether abortion ends an innocent life. That is where our political strategy needs to start, not end."

On a recent stormy day, when seeing a woman for a prenatal visit, I was reminded of the premier bill that many in the pro-life movement have fought for in recent years: The Pain Capable Unborn Child Protection Act. It essentially bans abortions after twenty weeks fetal development, claiming that as the marker for when babies in the womb can feel pain. (Additionally, the bill also aligns with current public opinion about the stage at which abortions should be banned.) Here's the problem. This woman I was serving in my capacity as an OB/GYN was carrying a baby at ten weeks gestational age. Outside, a bolt of lightning struck not far from the clinic—and, on the ultrasound, the baby visibly leaped at the piercing sound of thunder. It's a telling indicator that a baby has some capabilities with their five senses, and even pain receptors, far before twenty weeks. Haven't we had enough half-truths about human development codified into U.S. law already?

For those pro-life legislators (and nonprofit groups) committed to incremental strategies, there is one way their efforts may achieve some good. It is simply to *defend those pro-life laws* when they are challenged in state and federal courts. Spare no expense. Don't listen to lawyers who tell you about "unfavorable dynamics in the judicial pipeline" and get wrapped up in the balance of Left and Right on whatever court. No one knows what any given judge will decide when presented with the facts of a case. Therefore, ensure that the best medical and legal arguments are included in the evidence of your bill and defend it. Regarding the twenty-week abortion ban, it's a compelling argument that current U.S. law aligns our nation closely with the medical ethics of totalitarian states like North Korea and China. When well-written and defended vocally, even those incremental laws could set judicial precedents that elevate the child's rights.

How do we accomplish the laudable goal of achieving legislative and judicial recognition that human life begins at conception? Will U.S. law ever recognize that, once conceived, the child is entitled to the same protections to which all other human persons are entitled? The issue has certainly been made overly complex by the tortured logic that ignores science and fact. But the potential solutions are simple and straightforward. Do not misunderstand me—I did not say that it would be *easy*. By simple and straightforward, I mean that there are limited options to achieve redress—namely, two and only two.

Option one is probably the best but also the most difficult to achieve. It would be to create and ratify an amendment to the Constitution that recognizes that life begins at conception. Every human life, at each and every stage from conception to natural death, would be entitled under the equal protection doctrine of the Constitution to all the rights and liberties granted by the due process of law. It would enshrine in law that no person may have life or any other liberties taken from them. This is by far the most preferable, and such an amendment was proposed in the early 1970s soon after *Roe* was decided. However, it did not gain traction; it was opposed by abortion rights supporters within Congress, and it was not championed by those in Congress who claimed to be pro-life. Passage of an amendment to the Constitution of the United States is difficult, but it has been done twenty-seven times. It requires that a two-thirds majority of the House and of the Senate pass a proposed amendment, which must then be ratified by a majority of voters in two-thirds of the states. While difficult, it has been done before. While it is possible that such an amendment would be ratified by two-thirds of the states, there is currently an insurmountable obstacle in Congress. Specifically, the current number of Democratic members who support abortion rights and depend on Planned Parenthood donations is too great for that threshold to ever be achieved. Passage of a constitutional amendment of this kind would require a massive shift in electoral politics. The only other way a constitutional amendment can be passed is by a Convention of the States, and that has never been done.

That leaves us with the only other possibility—which is for state legislatures to craft legislation that incorporates personhood protections for the unborn. Such state laws can use justification drawn from the equal protection and due process doctrines of the Constitution, as well as drawing on natural law arguments, to create an opportunity for the Supreme Court to revisit the injustice of *Roe* and its bastard descendants. Achieving that goal will require a multi-faceted approach by grassroots activists. We must pressure legislative bodies and political figures, at the same time as policy-making bodies, professional lobbying groups, and special interest groups. Such a concerted effort will only be achieved by making an accurate understanding of life issues much more generally and widely known.

We must also be prepared for eventual victory. In the event that a constitutional amendment was ever passed, or *Roe* were to be reversed, it would bring several challenges to the forefront. The pro-life community would need to prove wrong the assertions that we are nothing more than "forced-birthers" who care little to nothing about the babies and the women once the child is delivered. We know this could not be further from the truth, but it has been a common accusation and will continue to be. We will need to continue to support pro-life pregnancy centers, as they currently do far more than show women the truth about abortion. They minister to the needs that these women and their children have, and will be called upon to do so in ever increasing numbers. Most of them are intimately connected with local adoption and foster care agencies, along with other child welfare advocacy groups. The need for pro-life convictions to be walked out will increase, not decrease, when *Roe* is cast upon the ash heap of history where it belongs.

It is my hope that this work has prepared and equipped the reader to defend the pro-life position with skill and confidence. Hopefully, you have become more aware of the vast array of opportunities and needs which exist in this battle. It is also my hope that some who may have seen the issue from a different point of view now can esteem life as it should be and stand ready to defend life at all its stages.

In conclusion, it should be said that pro-life convictions can be sufficiently defended on the basis of science, medicine, the law, general ethics, and morality. One can adequately make the case for defending life simply on the basis of human dignity, and in a secular society we must be able to do so. For those who are strongly pro-life and have no theological reason for being so, I welcome you and am glad to have you on our side. In our society, relying solely on theological arguments for issues such as this opens us to opposition from those with closed minds and should be avoided.

But for those of us who are grounded in the worldview that Christian theology brings, I would ask you to do one thing above all else—first and foremost in your pro-life efforts. Pray. Pray hard. Make the pro-life movement and the sanctity of life for our society a part of your daily prayer life. Prayer will not relieve you of being obligated to participate otherwise in whatever way you can. But it is, for those of us who call ourselves Christian, the starting point. Ask for wisdom, strength, and the ability to do that which you can, and petition God to do what only He can do.

We are at a critical point in human history, and the history of the United States. I believe the fight to save defenseless lives in the womb is the most important human rights issue of our time.

This is not some political issue or fleeting cause. My wife and I know firsthand the pain and guilt of seeing an innocent life lost too soon. We also know the healing forgiveness of our Heavenly Father whose love is perfect. Our prayer is that God would, in His providential power, protect life in all its stages. If experience is any guide, I believe He is going to use you and me to do it.

NOTES

1. Gallup, "Historical Trends on Abortion," https://news.gallup.com/poll/1576/abortion.aspx, accessed July 23, 2019.

2. Keith L. Moore, *The Developing Human: Clinically Oriented Embryology*, 2nd edition (Philadelphia, Penn: W. B. Saunders, 1977), 1.

3. Bradley M. Patten, *Human Embryology*, 3rd edition (New York, McGraw-Hill, 1968), 43.

4. Randy Alcorn, *Pro-Life Answers to Pro-Choice Arguments*, 2nd edition (Sisters, Oregon: Multnomah Publishers, 2000), 59.

5. Keith L. Moore, *The Developing Human: Clinically Oriented Embryology*, 2nd edition (Philadelphia, Penn: W. B. Saunders, 1977).

6. Bradley M. Patten, *Human Embryology*, 3rd edition (New York, McGraw-Hill, 1968).

7. Congress.gov, "S.311 - Born-Alive Abortion Survivors Protection Act," https://www.congress.gov/bill/116th-congress/senate-bill/311/all-actions, accessed July 23, 2019.

8. American Association of Pro-Life Obstetricians and Gynecologists, "References on Adverse Effects of Induced Abortion," https://aaplog.org/get-involved/references/, accessed July 26, 2019.

9. Adoption.com, "Infants for Adoption," https://adoption.com/infants-for-adoption, accessed July 26, 2019.

10. Randy Alcorn, *Pro-Life Answers to Pro-Choice Arguments*, 2nd edition (Sisters, Oregon: Multnomah Publishers, 2000)

11. Scott Klusendorf, *The Case for Life: Equipping Christians to Engage the Culture* (Wheaton, Illinois: Crossway, 2009)

12. Roland Warren, "Here's What A Man Should Say When Told To 'Shut Up' About Abortion," https://thefederalist.com/2018/03/17/heres-what-a-man-should-say-when-told-to-shut-up-about-abortion/, accessed July 28, 2019.

13. American Journal of Public Health, "Socioeconomic Outcomes of Women Who Receive and Women Who Are Denied Wanted Abortions in the United States," https://www.ncbi.nlm.nih.gov/pubmed/29345993, published March 2018.

14. Dr. John Patrick, "The Myth of Moral Neutrality," http://www.cmdscanada.org/my_folders/Resources/MythofMoralNeutrality.pdf, accessed July 28, 2019.

15. Congressional Research Service, "The Supreme Court's Overruling of Constitutional Precedent," https://fas.org/sgp/crs/misc/R45319.pdf, published September 24, 2018.

16. Gregory J. Roden, "Unborn children as constitutional persons," https://www.ncbi.nlm.nih.gov/pubmed/20443281, Issues in Law and Medicine, published spring 2010.

17. Texas Right to Life, "Kagan Writes ACOG Language against Partial-Birth Abortion," www.texasrighttolife.com/kagan-writes-ACOG-language-against-partial-birth-abortion/, accessed July 26, 2019.

18. The Christian Chronicle, "The church must break its 'Eerie Silence,'" http://christianchronicle.org/the-church-must-break-its-eerie-silence/, accessed July 26, 2019.

19. The Hill, "Anti-abortion Democrats fading from the scene," https:// thehill.com/homenews/campaign/345231-anti-abortion-democrats-fading-from-the-scene, published August 4, 2017.

20. NPR, "Abortion Vote Shows How Much Democrats' World Has Changed," https://www.npr.org/sections/itsallpolitics/2015/01/26/381472527/ abortion-vote-shows-how-much-democrats-world-has-changed, published January 26, 2015.

21. Fox News, "Progressive caucus co-chair calls for 'strong primary challenges' against anti-abortion Dems," https://www.foxnews.com/politics/ progressive-caucus-co-chair-calls-for-strong-primary-challenges-against-anti-abortion-dems, published May 18, 2019.

22. The Christian Post, "'Unplanned' was birthed by faithful prayer, says 40 Days for Life founder," https://www.christianpost.com/news/un-planned-birthed-faithful-prayer-40-days-for-life-founder.html, published March 27, 2019.

23. The Christian Post, "10 Reasons You Should Pray Outside an Abortion Center," https://www.christianpost.com/news/10-reasons-you-should-pray-outside-an-abortion-center.html, published March 13, 2015.

24. First Things, "Against Pro-Life Incrementalism," https://www.firstthings.com/web-exclusives/2019/05/against-pro-life-incrementalism, published May 23, 2019.

ACKNOWLEDGEMENTS

I must begin by thanking my Father in Heaven, for any talent or ability I have has ultimately come from Him.

I want to thank my wife, Julie. Without her, I would not be who I am today and would never have been able to complete this book. When asked how I am able to do the things I do, my frequent response is: "Because I have a great God and a great wife." Julie is a strong, brilliant, and beautiful woman. She has enriched my life more than I could ever have imagined anyone would.

The children Julie and I have raised have all been encouraging and supportive. Many thanks to Ashleigh, Alex, Austin, and Abigail.

My close friends Pastor Lyndon Allen, Joe Carr, and Dr. Omar Hamada have been invaluable. They have been fellow warriors, and have never failed to answer a call or text as I have worked through aspects of these issues. Lyndon's passion for advancing the Kingdom is contagious. Joe's knowledge of the history of the issue of abortion and his experience as a state legislator not only contributed to this book—he also was a significant part of my involvement in legislative efforts in my home state of Tennessee. Omar's training and experience as an obstetrician and the shared convictions we have are a source of strength.

Julie and I have enjoyed another wonderful friendship in Laura and Trent Messick. They have been on the front lines of the battle for life for almost forty years and were responsible for starting Murfreesboro's pro-life center, now known as Portico. They still lead there, and I have been blessed to serve as medical director in their ministry for more than ten years. Their wisdom and gentle manner, undergirded by fierce devotion, is an inspiration.

My editor, Josh Shepherd, has become a good friend. It has been a true act of providence for me to have found an editor as well-versed on the issues at stake. His skill has helped make this work a reality.

The team at NEWTYPE Publishing, especially Ryan Sprenger, Carmen Miller, and Chelsea Slade, have all exceeded my expectations, and they made it possible to get this book into your hands.

Our dear friend, Gwyn Miller, is an amazingly talented artist, and is responsible for the cover art. She made my mental vision a reality.

Finally, there are too many others to mention who supported my efforts with prayer and encouragement. These dear friends have my undying thanks.

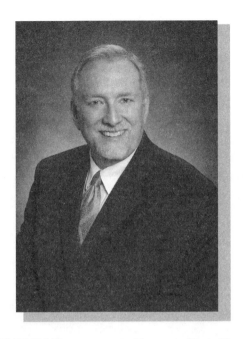

C. BRENT BOLES, M.D. grew up in Fountain Run, Kentucky on a farm raising beef cattle. For the past two decades, he has practiced medicine as an obstetrician/gynecologist (OB/GYN). A board-certified physician, he graduated from the University of Louisville School of Medicine.

Since residency, Dr. Boles has delivered approximately 7,000 babies into the world. Today, he serves families across central Tennessee through his medical practice at Covenant Healthcare for Women. He also currently has academic responsibilities as an assistant clinical professor for both the University of Tennessee Health Sciences Center Department of Emergency Medicine and the Meharry Medical College Department of Obstetrics and Gynecology.

In 2014, Dr. Boles became a volunteer spokesman for Yes on 1, a successful pro-life ballot initiative which amended the Tennessee state constitution. He is a member of the Christian Medical and Dental Associations as well as American Association of Pro-Life Obstetricians and Gynecologists.

Dr. Boles currently serves as medical director at Portico, a local pregnancy help center. He writes and speaks often on defending human life and dignity. Challenging popular pro-choice rhetoric, he applies principles of medical ethics to illuminate current issues.

He and his wife, Julie, live in Murfreesboro, Tennessee. They are parents of four children and now enjoy being grandparents of four (and counting).

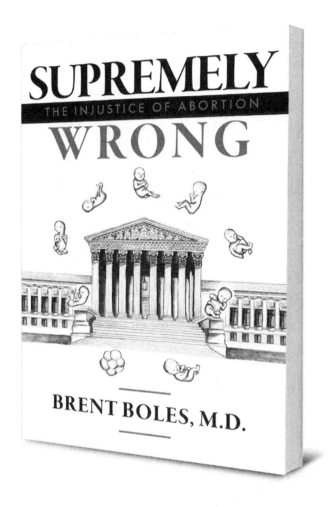

To order bulk copies of
Supremely Wrong,

Or to inquire about Dr. Brent Boles
speaking at your event,

Visit SupremelyWrong.com